Shared Governance
Implementation Manual

Shared Governance Implementation Manual

TIM PORTER-O'GRADY, EdD, RN, CS, CNAA, FAAN
Principal
Tim Porter-O'Grady, Inc.
Atlanta, Georgia

Illustrated

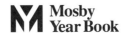

Mosby
Year Book

St. Louis   Baltimore   Boston   Chicago   London   Philadelphia   Sydney   Toronto

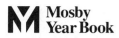
Mosby
Year Book
Dedicated to Publishing Excellence

Executive Editor: N. Darlene Como
Associate Developmental Editor: Brigitte Pocta
Project Manager: Peggy Fagen
Designer: Jeanne Wolfgeher

Printed in the United States of America.

Mosby-Year Book, Inc.
11830 Westline Industrial Drive
St. Louis, MO 63146

International Standard Book Number 0-8016-6317-2

97 CL/MY 9 8 7 6 5 4

Contents

Special Note

References to gender and the pronouns in this book are
often feminine. While the author recognizes that there are
nurses who are men, he also acknowledges that a large majority
of nurses are women and defers to that reality. In so doing, no
offense to either gender is implied or intended.

Introduction: Getting started with shared governance

This manual is meant to be a support "tool" for those interested in pursuing an organized effort to implement shared governance in their organization. While the focus is on the beginning phases of implementing a clinical model of shared governance, the process can be applied to any setting. Any one of the professions can use the information included in this workbook for implementing the shared governance concept in its unique setting.

This manual will be most useful when used in conjunction with the book, **Implementing Shared Governance: Creating a Professional Organization** (Mosby–Year Book, 1992). When used together, these two books provide a solid framework for effectively initiating the shared governance concept in any clinical service setting. Included in Appendix A of this book is an extensive bibliography of other resources that are helpful with specific components of implementing shared governance. For those looking for additional support, a number of facilities implementing shared governance have been identified in Appendix B. These facilities are committed to the process of shared governance and have in place resources to assist those who are interested in the developmental processes associated with implementing shared governance. The reader should be advised that some of these facilities offer implementation assistance as a part of their business operation and therefore may charge for their services. The subject of cost should be raised before asking for consultation or informational support from any facility listed in this manual.

The processes identified in this workbook are presented in a logical developmental sequence beginning with the concept of shared governance and ending with sample bylaws. Not all settings will require the information contained in every chapter. The book has been designed to facilitate broad use. Chapters that are of interest to the reader should be used as a support or for information, as required. Each chapter can stand alone and therefore can be used out of sequence with the others. The reader should be aware, however, that each chapter is essential to the process of implementation.

While this manual attempts to address the major implementation issues, it should not be used as a unilateral resource for implementation. It should be used in conjunction with other information resources. Together with other information, the reader will gain a comprehensive sense of the characteristics of implementation and how to achieve a successful shared governance organization.

Manuals and other documents that facilitate the developmental process are always in transition. The reader should evaluate the information contained herein with a critical eye; suggestions for improvements are welcomed. Please direct your suggestions to the publisher at the address listed on p. iv. Much of the success of shared governance has emerged because those implementing it were willing to share their experiences and to work diligently to improve the conditions and circumstances that support it. It is hoped that the reader's willingness to share will continue to enhance this manual and help refine it for future implementation of shared governance concepts.

It is also hoped that the implementation of shared governance concepts will be both an exciting and a personally rewarding process. It is a process involving constant transition and requires good judgment, patience, and commitment. The processes outlined in this manual may take varying lengths of time to implement. Each institution has its own unique variables that will influence how the process unfolds. Appendix E contains a sample implementation timeline that may be helpful to some readers. Sharing information and letting the process run its course are the two pieces of advice that will be most helpful in successfully implementing shared governance.

While this manual reflects 11 years of experience in the implementation of shared governance models, it is not conclusive. One of the dynamics of the implementation process is that more information is constantly becoming available as each setting learns something new about implementation and new models unfold. However, the principles of shared governance are consistent and have been incorporated in this manual (refer to Chapter 1 in **Implementing Shared Governance**).

The processes of implementing shared goverance are challenging. They demand major organizational and systems changes. However, they should also be fun. An organized and systematic approach to implementation provides an opportunity to write a script that facilitates the relationships among nurses and between nurses and others in the health care enterprise. It allows for large doses of humor, tears, good times, and challenge. Intense dialogue and controversy are characteristics of a major system change and should be expected (refer to Chapter 2 in **Implementing Shared Governance**).

Implementing shared governance is not a noiseless process. There will be many who will raise questions and demand responses, some who will not agree with the idea and fail to support it, and some who will grow to accept it as they come to understand what it means. Some of the leaders in the organization will be totally supportive of the efforts to empower the staff, while others will fight to see that it never happens. Most people will fall somewhere between these two extremes. All of this is a part of the dynamics of the implementation process and should be expected. Anything that creates as much potential for ownership and makes as much change as does shared governance cannot help but strike some significant chords in the organization and raise some important issues.

Shared governance often demands a willingness to build on trust and to create it when it is not present. There must be honesty in the organization that supports the effort. There can be no secrets in the implementation of shared governance. In fact, the opposite is true. As much information as is reasonable must be made available to the staff to support their involvement. This process alone increases the effectiveness and esprit de corps in the nursing organization. This will create challenge and raise questions, sometimes from unusual places, questions that demand open and honest responses.

It is hoped that this manual will be a valuable tool for those implementing shared governance. I hope that those who take the risk will be present to reap the rewards. The professions will change their roles and relationships within the health care system as each profession changes the places in which it does its work (not just at the national policy and professional level). It is in the places where staff practice their profession that change will be most meaningful and real. It is in these places where that change will also have the greatest impact. To the extent this manual helps in that process, it will have fulfilled its purpose.

Assessing the Individual's Perceptions

What is most important in moving toward shared governance is that there be a clear understanding about what it means to the individual and what it means to the institution. The reasons for interest in the process are many and varied. There is no single right reason or basis for interest. What is important is that the *real* reasons be clear and apparent to all involved. Honesty at the outset is the essential basis for exploring the values of shared governance and how they relate to the organization. The following personal and individual questions are helpful:

1. What do I want to know about shared governance?

2. What is my personal interest in shared governance? Why do I want it?

3. What frustrations do I see in my practice that raise questions about what currently is in place where I am?

4. How do I think my supervisor (boss) would respond to the thoughts I'm having about the organization?

5. Do I have a number of reasons not to like the way things are now:
   Am I angry?

   Am I burned out?

N   O   T   E   S

Am I disgusted?

Do I still like my work?

How do I think my colleagues feel?

Am I alone in these feelings?

How would shared governance address any of these issues? If it is something that I only have heard about, what is it that I think shared governance can do for my workplace?

QUESTIONS ABOUT THE ORGANIZATION

Often there is something about the place within which you work that creates a great deal of concern. Although many of the personal questions above can reveal this, sometimes it is better to think about the organization more objectively and identify those things that are of the most concern from your perspective. Taking time to write them helps formalize your thinking and give it clearer meaning:

The three things I most dislike about this workplace are:
      1.

      2.

      3.

The three things I most like about this workplace are:

    1.

    2.

    3.

My thoughts about my ability to do my work here are:

The staff is generally satisfied with working here except for:

The administration here is generally good but could be better if it:

I feel that I have been able to accomplish the following three things since I have been in this organization:

    1.

    2.

    3.

N   O   T   E   S

The goals I most wanted to be able to accomplish in my work but haven't been able to are:

1.

2.

3.

Assessing the Manager's Perceptions

THE MANAGER'S ROLE

Much of the success of shared governance depends on the perception and contribution of the managers at all levels of the organization. Indeed, shared governance cannot be successful if the management team is not in support of it. It is important that the perceptions of the manager and the application of the role in implementing shared governance be clarified and understood. The following questions related to the individual manager are helpful in clarifying individual perceptions of managers in the process of implementing shared governance.

CLINICAL OR SERVICE EXECUTIVE

The role of the service executive, whether a nurse or other professional executive, is vital in the design and implementation of shared governance. Because this workbook will be of benefit to all managers in any clinical service we shall identify the chief clinical administrator as a service executive. In all shared governance systems the executive (chief clinical officer) must be completely committed to the concept of shared governance and all that it implies. All too often the executive may give cursory support to shared governance at the outset only to modify his or her views and support when shared governance begins to make significant changes or creates more "noise" in the system than he or she anticipated or can accept. It is important that the executive be fully aware of what she is doing and committing to at the start so that later challenges do not shake the commitment and create difficulties from which it may be nearly impossible to recover.

The executive should ask himself or herself the following questions:

My predominant style of management is:

The following are the three most important factors influencing the role of the executive:

1.

2.

3.

The barriers in this organization to implementing shared governance are:

1.

2.

3.

Implementing shared governance in this organization will create the following major changes in this organization:

1.

2.

3.

4.

5.

The following peers in administration will have trouble with the notion of shared governance:

1.

Nature of his or her concern:

2.

Nature of his or her concern:

3.

Nature of his or her concern:

The executive will have to confront his or her peers with the reasons and purposes for creating a different organizational system. Since shared governance is accountability-based, he or she will have to be able to articulate the accountabilities and their impact on the organization. The five accountabilities for the professions are practice, quality assurance, education, research, and management. It is these accountabilities on which the concept of shared governance builds. The executive will have to be able to articulate them in an understandable way to his or her boss and colleagues in administration.

Important elements of the accountabilities affecting the service executive's belief system and implementation of shared governance are these: Practice (the work); Quality assurance (measurement); Education (assuring competence); Research (creation of new knowledge); and Management (resource control).

The executive must be willing to undergo personal change and change in the management team. Moving away from being the sole control and introducing control and authority to the staff is key to unfolding shared governance. Allowing that to happen means that a developmental program of personal and leadership change in the organization will be necessary. The executive will have to ask himself or herself the following questions:

How does the introduction of shared governance change my role as a nurse executive?

N O T E S

What three things will I have to change personally to make shared governance work in this setting? (*Refer to Chapter 5 in **Implementing Shared Governance.**)

  1.

  2.

  3.

What will be the most difficult behavior for me to change?

What is my plan for changing the above behavior? Action:

Evaluation:

Time frame:

What will my staff find in me that will be a major strength in making this change to shared governance?

What are the five expectations I have for shared governance from the perspective of the role of the executive?

  1.

  2.

3.

4.

5.

From the perspective of the executive what are the key changes in the management staff that would have to occur to facilitate a change to shared governance?

1.

2.

3.

Am I willing to undertake the activities and incur the risks of change to implement a shared governance system in my organization?

UNIT MANAGER

Perhaps the greatest support for shared governance will come from the unit manager. The problem here, however, is that the unit manager will undergo the greatest amount of the anticipated changes. This person will directly experience the empowerment and expanded role of the staff in decision making. In the service setting the unit manager will have to support the activities of shared governance that unfold at the unit level. At the outset the unit manager appears to have the most to lose as staff members increase their role in decisions made about their practice and professional lives.

The unit manager must be cognizant of the impact shared governance will have on him or her and the role of manager. A thorough understanding of the concept and some common principles on which shared governance is based is a good place to begin. To accomplish this, several personal developmental objectives need to be addressed:

1. Review personal/professional values
2. Establish a data base on shared governance
   library search
   literature review
   reading priorities
   generating information to peers
   discussion group with other managers
3. Question values and functions
4. Determine predominant management style
5. Unit plan for discussion of the concepts

The unit manager must be equally honest in self-analysis of beliefs and style and their impact on implementing shared governance. The most frequent problem experienced with implementing shared governance is the dissonance of the management team with regard to both the concept of shared governance and the successful transition of management behaviors necessary to support it.

The unit manager should ask himself or herself these questions:

What do I believe shared governance contributes to the health care organization?

   1.

   2.

   3.

How does the staff benefit in a shared governance organization?

   1.

   2.

   3.

What are the three greatest problems I have with the idea of shared governance?

1.

2.

3.

What is my plan for personal change with regard to those areas where there is conflict between my beliefs or management style and shared governance?

Goals?

Time line?

Evaluation?

Do I have a peer to whom I can relate regarding evaluation of my own changes in style and support?

Changing management style will be an important part of the transition in the role of the manager. Without some major shifts in the way in which the manager manages, there will be conflicts between the staff and the manager regarding authority and decision making. Therefore the manager must be aware of the kinds of changes required in the shared governance approach. These changes include:

> The manager will move from a directing role to a facilitating role. This means more asking, less telling; more supporting, less doing; more group work, less individual task assignment.

Staff will need permission to make decisions. Managers will have to be willing to accept the fact that good decisions may take time. A developmental approach to assisting good decision making will have to be planned by the manager as the staff acquires decision-making skills.

Some control issues will have to move to the staff. Those issues related to practice, quality of care, competence, and evaluation will have a greater staff role. The manager will have to be comfortable with this transition of accountabilities.

The manager will need to feel that his or her boss accepts these changes and that both of them support the changes and each other as they accommodate and lead the changes.

The manager will have to select some of the issues to move to the staff based on their preparedness, his or her personal comfort, and the degree of risk in the decision. Strategizing for success will be important.

Avoiding taking the more controlling and easy way to do things will be especially tough for the manager. At times when it would be more convenient to do something oneself, the manager will need to allow the staff to make the decision. This sometimes calls for extreme patience.

More personal questions for the manager in getting ready for implementing shared governance include:

What causes me to exercise the control that may prevent me from allowing the staff to do something I know I could do better and faster?

Over what kind of issues could I reasonably begin to let the staff assume more control?

1.

2.

3.

What are the three most likely responses I will have when I see the staff making decisions I have problems with?

    1.

    2.

    3.

Are they appropriate?

If my reactions are not appropriate, what will I do when I see them surfacing?

Do I have a "fall back" strategy if staff don't appear to be moving in the right direction or even moving at all?

    The leadership roles of the executive and the management team are vital to the success of the shared governance approach. Shared governance has never succeeded anywhere if the management team has not supported it. Support means the willingness to undergo personal and professional change and to lead that change in the staff. A great deal of commitment is required to do that. The nurse manager must be sensitive to the impact of change on himself or herself and relationships with the staff, as well as his or her expression of the management role. As Table 1 indicates, there is a transition from focus on the self to focus on group relationships and functions. The manager must be able to provide an environment that emphasizes the group or team values and processes.

TABLE 1
From Motivation to Empowerment

1960s-1970s	1980s-1990s
Focus on self	Begin with self
Isolation of work and self	Concert of work and self
Motivation of self and others	Group integration and value
Personal growth and work outcomes	Empowerment—group and work well-being
Conflict resolution strategies	Integration/ownership and stakeholding

The manager must be able to seek and get support in this transition. He or she must count on the support of the person to whom he or she reports and the support and encouragement of peers. The executive plays the largest role in providing the initial support and firm commitment to movement to shared governance. Any wavering in that commitment on the executive's part can be easily seen by the managers and the staff and creates a tenuousness in the process which may compromise the energy necessary to make it work. This confidence that it is appropriate and right for the organization must be presence at the outset.

Leadership is primarily inspiration and secondarily perspiration. Success is more a matter of relationship than function. As an organization goes through a great deal of change, as suggested by shared governance, the connection between the managers and the executive will be important. The model of that relationship serves as a framework for the emerging relationship in the staff. Trust and dependence on each other in the process of implementation will be vital.

All initial efforts in exploring the shared governance process are in understanding the concept and in building a common understanding regarding what it means. Time for this must be provided first for the managers. Only then can it move to the staff. Problems and issues with the managers' understanding and role need attention at the outset so that some common basis for implementation can be assured.

It should be anticipated that the concept of shared governance raises a lot of important personal and professional issues with the management team. Time in working out these issues is essential if a strong premise and foundation for shared governance are to be in place. Knowledge is only one of the conditions necessary to successful implementation. Personal feelings, insights, fears, and perceptions are as important in the process of successful implementation and can be as critical in preventing it from happening in the organization.

Assessing the Staff's Perceptions

The most challenging part of implementing shared governance is the activities related to involving the staff and changing their perceptions about decision making and their role in it (see Chapter 5 in **Implementing Shared Governance**). Exploring staff feelings about their current circumstances and their desire for change is an important part of the move to implementing shared governance.

The first questions that are important to staff are those relating to staff satisfaction with the workplace and specific perceptions related to that satisfaction. Two very useful and effective research instruments (included in Appendix C) are the Stichler Collaborative Behavior Scale (CBS), developed by Jaynelle F. Stichler, and the Nurse Opinion Questionnaire (NOQ), developed by Ruth Ludemann and the Nursing Research Committee at Rose Medical Center in Denver, Colorado.

Another valuable tool is David Allen's "Shared Governance Evaluation Instrument." It is very user friendly, making it a highly useful tool. Both tools can be used for transitional analysis and should be administered once a year at the same time to the same groups originating the study for the duration of the implementation period (see Appendix C for David Allen's instrument).

In addition to the above instruments, the following questions are important to the staff involved in implementing shared governance:

I understand the concept of shared governance fully?
Yes   No

If no, the three main parts I do not understand are:
     1.

     2.

     3.

N O T E S

If yes, I like the concept and feel ready to move ahead with it.
Yes   Except for:

I think my colleagues feel the same way I do.
Yes   No

If no, my reasons for thinking this are:
  1.

  2.

  3.

What are the three most important things I would want the shared governance approach to do for me?
  1.

  2.

  3.

If I could freely say what I most want from my profession, what would be the two most important things to me?
  1.

  2.

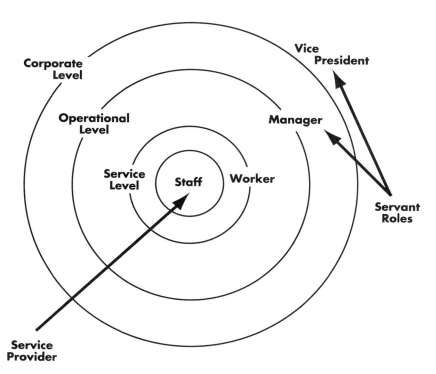

FIGURE 3-1
The organic model for the 21st century health care organization.

If I could freely say, what would be the two most important things I would want from my organization?

1.

2.

INFORMATION NEEDS

If the staff is to be able to do anything meaningful related to shared governance, they must have access to as much data as possible regarding the shared governance process. The planner, however, should not be concerned if the staff members do not appear to be highly interested in the concept in the beginning. They will not be interested in understanding or implementing something that does not appear, at the outset, to affect their lives in a very meaningful way. It will take some time before that changes, and the implementors should be very patient.

Do not undertake a broad-based, service-wide education program for the staff regarding implementing shared governance. To implement an expensive, time-consuming staff education program before the staff is ready to learn is a waste of time and money. People do not learn what they are not ready to hear. Learning occurs best when the material learned directly affects individual lives or can be immediately applied in ways that make a difference to the individual.

Make information available to those interested. Get them more involved. Trust the implementation process and take the time necessary to let individuals lead peers into broadening the peers' interest in what is going on. Make sure that literature and other information are readily available at the unit level and that questions raised can be addressed in a knowledgeable way in a relatively short time.

The following topics should be included in the available literature on the unit:

Professional roles
Participatory management
Changes occurring in health care
Brief history of professions
Shared governance concepts
Shared governance models

(See suggested references in Appendix A.)

Specific needs of the staff related to issues of shared governance should be accommodated to the extent possible. A central data base should be available where new or interesting additions to the information available can be retained and accessed by interested staff. Information specific to new organization designs that are more "organic" in structure, as shown in Figure 3-1, reflect an entirely new approach to the workplace and should be emphasized in researching shared governance. Note that the pyramidal structure symbolic of the bureaucratic model is replaced with concentric circles representing a more democratic, less authoritarian approach.

The following questions will help staff members focus on their own informational needs as they explore their initial interest in shared governance:

How do I think management feels about this concept?

What does the current organization find most threatening about shared governance?

    1.

    2.

    3.

What does it take to really make shared governance successful?

What changes would I have to make:
      in my practice?

      in my relationships?

      in my beliefs about work?

      in my contribution to shared governance?

What is the single most important change I would have to make in a shared governance organization?
      1.

Do I really want this kind of change?
      Does my manager?

      Do my peers?

How will the hospital change if we implement shared governance?

How will hospital administration have to change to support this concept?

<u>N   O   T   E   S</u>

What do I still wish I knew more about related to shared governance?

1.

2.

3.

Beginning Implementation

THE TASK FORCE

Implementation of shared governance must begin with a thorough understanding of the concept and implications (see Chapter 2 in **Implementing Shared Governance**). The personnel requiring the most knowledge at the outset are the nurse executive, his or her associates, and the initial leadership group involved in exploration and initiation of implementation.

The initial task force is not the group who will be charged with the responsibility of implementation. They will start to put together the initial structures out of which the shared governance process will unfold. A very careful period of discernment between management and staff leadership with regard to the concept and its implementation in the organization is imperative. The task force does this initial exploration.

The task force should be formed from the creative, innovative, and risk-taking individuals of the organization. Because this could describe a whole host of persons, it is wise to select those who have the time, energy, and interest in shared governance. This group should be relatively broadly based and represent all forums in the department or service. It should not be too large a group but relatively representative of the kinds of professional resources of the staff. It should be comprised, where possible, of at least the following:

Service executive
1 Associate administrator/director
2 Unit managers
1 Clinical specialist or expert (if available)
1 Clinical educator
5 or 6 Staff members

The reader should note that representation between staff and others is relatively equal. It is important at the outset to make a statement about equity in membership of groups and the role of the staff in decisions that affect their future. Creating matching membership by equating staff members to other roles is a good first step. At first, the dialogue between staff and others may be tenuous and slow, but it usually improves as staff achieves comfort in exploring concepts and processes that may have not been open to staff discussion in the past.

The following are common activities of the task force:

1. Exploring the concept of shared governance and contrasting it with current activities in the organization
2. Moving toward some common understanding of what shared governance is and its relationship to professional practice

3. Anticipating potential problems in the organization with regard to implementing shared governance and their impact on it
4. Exploring feelings in the group about readiness and meaning to the organization related to implementing shared governance
5. Making the initial decision to implement shared governance and form the framework for the Shared Governance Coordinating Council (or steering committee)

In this group the initial issues and concerns are raised. Here the information is gathered, explored, and generated to the staff. Dialogue, controversy, input from a wide variety of sources, debate, discussion and problem solving characterize this time period and are inherent in this group's work in implementing shared governance.

The work of the task force is a significant undertaking. The initial commitment of the organization usually sets it on a path from which it is very difficult to retreat once the process has been initiated. It promises a great deal to the profession and the individual members of the management and staff. It is very difficult to stop this kind of implementation since its goal is to transform the organization. It is a commitment that should not be taken lightly.

It is required that the clinical executive formally and publicly commit to shared governance before implementation begins at any level of the organization. There will be some tough times and a strong need for perseverance and commitment at times when it might seem easier to move away from it. It is important that certain symbolic demarcations be noted. The clinical or service executives' formal commitment is one of them. Without it, the process will never be successful.

Resources required

The role of the task force should focus on providing an appropriate basis for beginning implementation of shared governance. Primary among their considerations is the availability of the resources necessary for the implementation process. The following resources should be secured by the task force before proceeding to form the steering process for shared governance implementation.

_____ Adequate shared governance literature
_____ Documented support from the Nurse Executive
_____ Sufficient people to begin implementation
_____ Management leadership understanding of shared governance
_____ No major staffing problem
_____ Willingness to do the work
_____ Financial resources to support implementation

The above guidelines influence the beginning of the process and should be addressed before the shared governance implementation begins. This transformational work will need as many supports in place as possible. Taking care of these basics will provide a firm basis on which to start the process.

THE SHARED GOVERNANCE COORDINATING COUNCIL (SGCC) OR STEERING COMMITTEE

The shared governance coordinating council (referred to as the SGCC) or steering committee is the first major group to undertake work regarding implementing shared governance. This group is empowered to control and manage the initial implementation process associated with creating a shared governance organizational model.

The most important initial factor influencing this group is the selection of members. There has been a great deal of discussion regarding how to put this group together in an appropriate manner. It appears, however, that how the group is constructed at the outset is less important than who makes up the membership. While a democratic selection process feels better to the organization, there is no evidence that it is the most effective method of selection. The important point is that the SGCC membership be such that the diversity, ability, and commitment be sufficient to undertake the work of creating and managing the implementation of the process.

The task force usually participates in determining the selection process for the SGCC. Sometimes members of the task force become members of the SGCC. This works to the extent that such transition is representative of the staff as a whole.

Some guidelines to assist in forming the SGCC are:

1. The SGCC should represent the staff as a whole.
2. The SGCC should not be larger than 14 members; the best working size ranges from 7 to 10 members.
3. The SGCC should have at least the following representation:
   A majority of staff nurses
   Nurse executive and/or designate
   A clinical specialist (if available)
   A unit manager(s)
4. There needs to be a regular meeting time at least once a month for a minimum of 2 hours each session, more at the outset.
5. Members must want to be there and remember that they are writing a script for the profession at their facility, not simply for their individual departments or units.

Selection process

The following questions help the task force pull together the initial coordinating council membership:

How many services are present in the organization?
Depending on the hospital size, the SGCC may represent major services (in hospitals over 150 beds) or units (in hospitals under 150 beds). In nonhospital settings there should be at least one representative for every 50 to 75 full-time equivalents. The goal is to keep membership size below 14 members.

Identify the services or units represented.

List the non-nurse positions on the SGCC.

Are there any people who should be considered for membership for political reasons?

Is there someone in the organization who should be a member because of his or her unique expertise?

What is the anticipated start date for the coordinating council?

Empowerment

When the work of selection is complete, the shared governance coordinating council begins its work. This group is the essential first step in putting form to the shared governance process. It is the first vestige of a governance group empowered with authority to make specific and key decisions with regard to the future structure of the clinical organization.

Formal empowerment of this group is essential if it is to willingly and confidently undertake its task. For this reason it is advised that the executive or designate (preference is always that the executive person have personal membership in order to deliver a message of highest level commitment and support) be a permanent member of the SGCC.

The formal powers of this group to transform the service structure and organization are formidable. Needless to say, if a new script is to be written for the organization, this group must have the ability and resources, as well as power, to undertake this work. The following powers must be defined and clarified as a part of the structuring of the SGCC to do its work:

1. The ability to define its own operating rules and regulations regarding:
   meeting times
   membership tenure
   method of decision making
   powers
   resource needs (budget and consultants)
   accountabilities of members
   time frames
2. The definition of the powers of the chairperson to:
   call the meeting
   control the agenda
   move the group to decision making
   remove nonparticipating members
   make group assignments
   accept no personal assignments
   speak for the SGCC between regularly scheduled meetings

Defining the role and rules for the chair is perhaps the most important initial task for the SGCC. The chair must have the freedom to undertake the role with the attendant governance powers that accrue to the role. This person's role is to see that the SGCC does its work and that each member contributes to it to the fullest extent possible. In this context the chairperson can move the group to make decisions, remove nonparticipating members, and make assignments. The following questions should be considered when electing the chairperson:

Who should be eligible?

Usually the chair of a shared governance SGCC is selected from among the staff members of the SGCC. However, issues of ability, skills, and preparation

How long should the chairperson serve?

Service is usually computed in the same manner that membership on the SGCC is determined. Sometimes, for continuity, groups may choose to have the chairperson serve for a longer term.

3. The purposes and time frames for completing the work of the SGCC. This group establishes the implementation plan for shared governance and must therefore have the essential components of the plan clearly in place and evaluate progress against expectations. It is clear that this initial plan will not likely look like what eventually takes shape but it does guide the thinking and implementation processes as the plan unfolds.

4. The ability to deal with issues impacting implementation of shared governance as they arise. It is certain that the work is not going to cease during the implementation of a new organizational model. A forum for making operational decisions must be incorporated into the thinking of the group as it puts together newer structures for problem solving.

5. A safe forum for dealing with the hard issues of governance and operating relationships. There must be a safe place where frank and open discussions affecting the organization and the implementation of shared governance get addressed. Ambiguity is the enemy of shared governance. Unresolved issues, hidden agendas, personal biases left unaddressed, incomplete patterns of planning, unexpressed concerns, and so on will intercept effective planning and implementation. When not dealt with they have a way of impeding progress and creating great problems in implementation.

Setting up the SGCC to be effective is the most important initial work of the SGCC. Commitment here will pay off in the effectiveness of the implementation process. Honest, open dialogue in the SGCC sets the stage for dealing with all the political and relational aspects affecting successful implementation. There must be commitment to openness and the ability to deal with real issues affecting the organization. Secrets, hidden agendas, boundary setting, nonnegotiables, and so on contribute to diminishing the effectiveness of the process.

The following questions help the members of the SGCC understand their initial commitments:

How will I best represent those who selected me?

What role do I expect to play in the development of shared governance?

What does being a member of the SGCC mean to me?

What are the time commitments of the role?

Do I need leadership development for this role and how do I identify those deficits for which I will need learning?

Am I ready to deal with real issues and do I agree to openly deal with those issues that concern me in a nonpassive and nonaggressive manner?

Am I willing to do "homework," reading, and some shared governance functions on nonwork time?

What do I think will be my personal impediment to effective membership on the SGCC?

What is my primary obligation to my peers who are also members of the SGCC?

Although these are not all the questions that should be asked by the new member of the SGCC, they are some of the most important (see Appendix D). As indicated, the degree of commitment to writing the new script for the organization is time consuming but significant. Each of the members must recognize this at the outset of the council's work and make some important decisions in the beginning, not later in the process when that member's role may be more important to the other members.

Sound membership on the SGCC is vital to the successful initiation of the shared governance process. Members will be expected to participate fully in decisions that affect the future and the design of the shared governance model. Therefore care should be exercised when selecting members. Because the rules of the workplace operating at the time of consideration of shared governance take precedence, whatever mechanism that works is the one of choice for the initial selection of these key people. Keep in mind that cross-sectional representation with a preponderance of staff will be the most desirable format for membership in this group.

Meetings

Important to the process of implementation is the structuring of the work and the initiation of meetings and the rules, regulations, and guidelines that make meetings effective. In many professional organizations, meetings are rampant without outcomes to justify their frequency. In shared governance the structure of meetings is vital to the work itself.

The following activities are essential to the beginning phases of the SGCC's work:

1. Establish the goals of the SGCC at the outset. The members should know what their purpose and objectives are for the work that the SGCC will be undertaking. Clarity of purpose at the inception of its work will facilitate the process of implementation.

2. Define the meeting times at the beginning so that long-range planning can be incorporated into the members' schedules. This is governance work for the profession in the institution; members should not miss meetings because of other obligations or time constraints.

3. Make clear role assignments so that expectations for participation and membership can be easily understood. Ambiguous expectations ensure that outcomes will not be achieved.

4. Governance work is the profession's work inside the organizational system. It should be expected that it is paid time and that time at work should be provided for governance activities.

5. The decisional process should be clear to the members. How discussion will unfold, the expectations for participation and dialogue, and the trust-building process associated with creating the group's own culture should be explored with members. Sometimes it is good to have an educator or group specialist help the group develop the kinds of skills necessary to be an effective group.

6. The group should be clear about its mandate and be free to pursue its objectives. The senior manager in the service should be present or a member of this group and indicate in the clearest terms his or her support for the concept and involvement in the process. *Shared governance never works if the senior management is not in support of it.*

THE WORK OF THE SGCC

Whatever other objectives the SGCC might construct for itself, it must at least be directed to exploring the shared governance concept and its implications, deciding on a model, devising an implementation plan, and evaluating the process. Since it is a group not likely to exist beyond the need for it, the SGCC should also have a good notion of the time for its termination in the implementation process. This is a transitional team. Planning therefore should include those structures in the model that will replace the SGCC.

All the processes associated with planning should be couched within the context of a time frame. Time serves the purpose of providing points of measure or a demarcation along the way that furnishes opportunities to evaluate progress. *No goals should be set without planning a time frame associated with their completion.*

Initial activity of the SGCC relates to itself first, as identified above. Work related to the implementation of shared governance itself is also first on the agenda. The culture of shared governance actually begins with this group and is then generated throughout the whole organization.

Some implementors will be concerned at this point about the unit level involvement in shared governance and will no doubt be raising questions about its initiation at the unit level. As indicated in the text **Implementing Shared Governance,** development at the unit level should proceed *following* the establishment of the professional direction for it in the division as a whole. Since shared governance is a professional model that advances the interests of the profession and its members in the best interests of patient care, the principles and premises on which the profession will build shared governance should be clearly established first.

Establishing the principles of shared governance assists the clinical organization to build a shared governance approach that is consistent and integrated and works in a way that benefits both the organization and the profession. Often, when development merely reflects the unit culture and values without a prevailing consistent overlay in the division as a whole, the work units fail to represent a consistent core of values that allow them to talk to each other, or represent the professionally delineated framework for shared governance (that is represented in Figure 4-1).

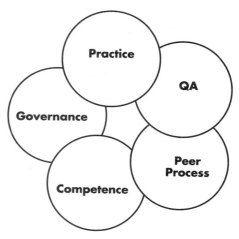

FIGURE 4-1
Structural integration for the professional organization.

Instead they sometimes subjugate their broad perspective of their profession to their unique and individual needs. In many ways they do this differently on each unit and no expression of a core framework is ever achieved. If the units have been implementing long enough, even their individual concepts and values associated with shared governance are so different that they may not be able to communicate with each other for lack of a common base of understanding. It must be remembered that shared governance is not designed simply to satisfy only the individual worker (which it does), but more importantly to advance the profession in the work setting and to improve the access to and delivery of health care to those who benefit from health services.

This reality is important to the initiation of the SGCC's work. They can begin the process with a broad-based focus without necessarily limiting the energy and drive of individual units that are anxious to increase the involvement of their staff in shared decision making. It is important to realize that individual work units can begin efforts at collaborative problem solving and structuring without waiting for the SGCC to tell it what to do. Indeed many shared governance approaches have begun just this way. The point that must be kept in mind is that the structuring of shared governance consistent with the goals of the profession in the service setting at any level must be driven by the professional body as a whole. That "corporate" structure must depend on the ability of the unit to fit that framework to a defined degree and thereby to exemplify in their unit structure the values determined appropriate by the SGCC. Each institution will have to manage this tension and determine how to keep unit problem solving and shared governance design operationally consistent with the beliefs essential to all nurses in the service setting. The SGCC should help minimize the ambiguity and the emergence of disparate activities at the unit level.

Responsibilities of the chair

Development of the chair is an important part of the process of moving toward shared governance. Since the chair should most often be selected from among the staff members of the SGCC, it is likely that the person will not have the kinds of leadership skills that are necessary for such a formidable task. The role of the administrative person on the SGCC helps to provide both role modeling and insights into the process of group leadership. Often, it is helpful for the chair of the SGCC and the senior nurse manager on the group to meet before meetings to strategize the chair's role and the management of the agenda or critical issues or processes that frequently arise during group work.

Leadership development attention generally relates to the following skills:

group management
Robert's Rules
conflict resolution
setting agenda priorities
individual problem members
task assignment
solution seeking
facilitation of group members
setting objectives, determining outcomes
speaking and communication skills

Questions related to the above that the chair may need to consider at the outset are:

1. With which of the above expectations am I most comfortable?
   Least comfortable?

2. How will I go about learning what I need to know in those areas I am unsure about?

3. Are there mentors or role models I can depend on to assist in my leadership development?

4. What am I most uncertain about in assuming the role of chair?

5. What assurances do I need to have to be successful in this role?

6. How will I take care of my needs in this position to keep me in balance?

7. Who in the group (SGCC) will act as my validator on whom I can depend to be open and honest with me when I need feedback and/or support?

The chairperson's role is very important at the outset of this process. She perhaps best represents the expression of empowerment in the staff. Careful selection and development of this chair can make the transition to shared governance much smoother and better received.

The relationship of the executive with this role is important, too. Validation of its importance can be evidenced in the nurse executive acting as role model and partner with the chair in the process of implementing shared governance. This relationship can be the best evidence of the organization's commitment to the implementation process. In this relationship the dialogue necessary for problem solving, political awareness, mutuality, and support can provide some of the strongest underpinnings for building successful shared governance.

Selecting a model

Becoming informed is always the first step. Shared governance has been in place in health care facilities for 11 years now. There is a growing body of knowledge in the area that can provide a great deal of assistance in understanding the concept. The SGCC must make sure that its members know enough about the concept to be able to make some knowledgeable decisions about what direction to move in its implementation. In Appendix B of this workbook are the names of some of the institutions around the country that are in some stage of successful implementation. Between the literature and the facility resources, the SGCC should be able to find ample data and supporting information to provide a foundation of knowledge for decisions related to implementation.

This information should provide ample material to assist in model selection and the development of a transitional plan (also see Chapter 4 in **Implementing Shared Governance**). Some issues that the information and knowledge building should address are:

1. Kinds of model designs available for consideration
2. Problems and opportunities in implementation
3. Values exemplified in the models
4. Consistency of principles with model design
5. Integration of models with the values of shared governance
6. Degree of empowerment of the staff
7. Distance of the model's design from the bureaucratic or institutional hierarchical structures
8. Well-integrated formal structures
9. Relationship established between unit and divisional structure
10. Representational basis of any of the designs

In addition to the above issues, the SGCC members should raise the following questions about what they read and hear:

How well are the models presented? Are they understandable?

Which models appear most thoroughly developed?

Are there good data to support model presentations?

Do they appear staff driven? Management driven?

Do you have a better "feel" for a particular model?

How do the models compare to your own culture?

What are some of the models' greatest shortcomings? (They all have some!)

Are you clear on what you want from shared governance?

The above questions are just some of the basic issues that the SGCC will have to consider. The culture and values of each setting will influence the formation of other questions and issues.

The matter of fit is very important. *There is no one best model*. The key for evaluating every model is its consistency with any of the principles on which shared governance is built. In many cases the SGCC may choose to select elements from a variety of models and fit the elements with their own institutional culture or specific intentions.

Some SGCC groups like to select a couple of models or approaches that best appeal to them. As a part of discerning their response they may present each to the staff or leadership from staff and management to gain valuable insights regarding the models' impact on the staff. Frequently staff and management from outside the group can clarify thinking regarding the fit of one model or another with the perceptions they share with the SGCC.

When the SGCC looks at the various models and opens dialogue for approaches related to implementation, it is important that they discuss the best way to get started in the implementation process. There are several points of view with regard to the best approach. The choice of which approach is best for the individual institution is driven by their culture and operational characteristics.

The methods most often chosen relate to either a division-wide approach or a pilot approach. If an organization is in good operational "health;" that is, has few financial or personnel problems, a division-wide implementation process is always desirable. This approach allows all to initiate the process, makes the initiation a professional strategy, builds internal supports and consultation, and assures organizational integration. The oldest, most successful models in the United States were developed division-wide and implemented at one time.

Since there is a wide variety of levels of integration in many organizations, this approach may not be possible. Using pilot approaches can be very helpful to those who either are tentative regarding the process or have some organizational limitations that do not permit them to generalize the implementation effort. *It should be clear, however, that implementation at the divisional level will be essential if shared governance as a professional model is to be fully successful.* How one moves in that direction is an issue of strategy that will reflect the values and culture of the organization implementing shared governance. The following questions will be helpful in determining which strategy is the best for the individual service setting:

Is there broad-based support and commitment from the entire division (department) for implementing shared governance?

Is the majority of energy for implementing shared governance coming from a few service units?

How broad is the understanding of the shared governance concept?

Is the clinical services division (or nursing) highly decentralized or incorporated into a product or service line format?

Where is most of the encouragement for implementing shared governance originating?

Is shared governance included in the division's strategic plan?
Yes   No

Are most of the goals of shared governance related to unit objectives or to the division's (department's) objectives?

Are there budget problems in the division (department)?

Are there staffing problems in the division (department) that have yet to be resolved?

What is the trust level in the division (department) or unit?

Is the prevailing view of the SGCC that it should be a division-(department-)wide program or initially unit based?

As previously indicated, the concept can be initiated in a number of ways. Since it is a professional model that organizes decision making into an effective operating framework, there must be a point when it affects the work of the profession as a whole in some fundamental ways. To do so indicates that it must represent all of the service in a structure that integrates its various departments, lines, and units or components in an integrated structure.

The major danger in the approach that has shared governance implemented in the entire service is the risk involved in such a wholesale implementation approach. The dangers related to impact on other services and the medical staff, the potential for large scale failure, and the tremendous degree of change that is thrust on the service can be very threatening and intimidating.

The danger in the pilot approach relates to the acculturation of implementation, which ensures that models reflecting one unit's value system and approach do not always translate to another. Also, the incidence of elitism is increased in settings that use this method with all the envy and passive aggressiveness that accompany it. The danger that the model chosen at the unit level will not replicate in other settings or units is accelerated and increases that chance that it fails to make a significant impact on the role and relationship of the profession to the delivery of health care services.

Clearly the issue of approach is very important to the appropriate implementation of the shared governance system. The answer to the above questions will determine the method of implementation and influence the outcome of the work and the design of the model. It must be very carefully considered.

Implementing the Governance Councils

The approach of this workbook is the implementation of shared governance within the entire division (department) rather than within a single unit of service. Also, the councilor model is used as the framework for implementation simply because it is the single most frequently developed model in the United States and there are more data available regarding its implementation. However, the rules and guidelines for implementation are the same for any of the models. The adjustments are more related to focus than to substance. The strategies for implementation included in this section are appropriate for any of the models. The reader need only substitute his/her design for the one identified here.

Figure 5-1 depicts the councilor model.

DEVELOPMENT OF A PLAN

As with any major change, it is appropriate to develop a strategy for implementation to serve as a map to the implementors and a tool for evaluation. Since what we achieve rarely looks exactly like what we conceive, the planners should expect differences in outcomes from those originally planned. At the outset it is often difficult to see the outcome of one's work with the same clarity of vision one has after having achieved success. The process teaches us much about what we have done that could have been learned only by doing it. This especially holds true in the implementation of shared governance.

This section is meant as a guide only. Not every element that the implementors of shared governance confront can possibly be anticipated. The major components of the process, however, are covered here and will serve as an appropriate backdrop to individual program planning.

The plan really has two parallel implementation patterns: one for the managers and the other for the clinical staff. Since so much adjustment must be undertaken in the role of the manager, it becomes imperative at the outset that the manager be the focus of attention in the planning process as soon as possible. It should be anticipated that the planning time line will be a minimum of 3 years. The organization is undergoing significant organizational change—indeed, transformation—and that cannot be accomplished overnight. The anticipated time for full implementation is from 3 to 5 years. This does not mean that it takes this long to see organizational and behavioral change (this happens soon after the first year), but it does mean that it takes a considerable amount of time for the process to be completed.

THE ROLE OF MANAGEMENT

The first year for the management team is critical to the success of the process. Most of the initial work with the management is developmental in nature. This

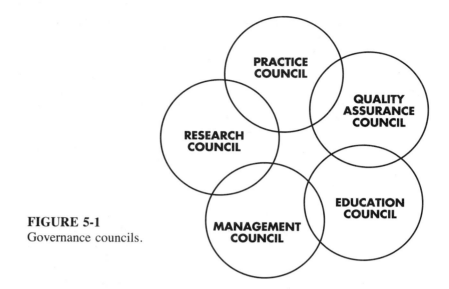

FIGURE 5-1
Governance councils.

means that understanding, accepting, and leading the process is essential to the success of shared governance. Many of the behaviors that lead to success in shared governance are idealized in the industrial models but rarely actualized. If shared governance is to be successful, these behaviors will have to emerge in the manager's role (see Appendix E).

The shift in accountability for the issues of practice, quality assurance, education, and research toward the staff's role also changes the role and relationship of the manager and calls for some developmental work that will assist the manager in understanding and facilitating her emerging role and the authority of the professional staff.

Issues related to the first year of management development include:

Introduction to the concept of shared governance
Management values clarification in shared governance
Impact of shared governance on accountability
Changes in authority in shared governance
Increased role of the staff in shared governance
Systems model design and impact on the role of the manager

The role of the manager in shared governance becomes a serious area of dialogue. Since the growth of the staff is essential to the successful implementation of shared governance, the manager must be able to move successfully from the role of director to facilitator. She knows that the staff must have a role in decision making consistent with their area of accountability.

The unit manager must be aware of the areas of accountability that are hers and her expected performance within them. The five areas of management accountability that are central to the role of the manager are:

Human resource provision
Fiscal resources (dollars and budgets)
Material resources
Support activities
Systems management

The manager must be able to exemplify the skills necessary to effectively perform the role of manager. There is often a great deal of debate about whether the clinical manager is primarily a coordinator of clinical care or a part of the organi-

TABLE 5-1

Differences Between the Management Team and the Management Council

Management Team	Management Council
Usually controlled and run by the clinical or service executive	Made up of all levels of management
Can make recommendations or participate in policy recommendations for approval of the executive	Sets policy and direction within the management accountability. Has a defined obligation to make decisions
Is usually formed for discussion and to make suggestions to the formal manager(s)	Is an accountability-based body with clear authority
Often limited to those at the "top" of the clinical organization	Clinical or service executive is a member with a defined role and single vote in decisions made by the group
Is not invested with formal powers and authority	In many cases in larger organizations is an elected group representing the interests of their management peers

zation and the management team. In shared governance the controversy is resolved. The clinical manager is defined by the manager role, not by staff or clinical delineations. Since role definition, not status or positioning on the hierarchy, is central to effectiveness in shared governance, the manager holds an equitable position with the staff. However, it is described in a different context from the practicing or clinical professional. The role is important, valuable, and necessary to shared governance. Only its characterization and expectations change.

The role of the manager is defined within the five basic accountabilities of management as identified by Mintzberg (see earlier discussion). These role characteristics can be identified as central to the expectations of the role of manager. Skill becomes critical to the exercise of the manager's role, and a certainty regarding the manager's ability to exercise this skill is vital, especially in a system of shared accountability. Each of the players must be able to play his or her assigned role effectively. All other roles depend on the ability of each player to do his or her part. The essential skills are not often identified, however.

If the manager is to exemplify the essential skills, she must know what they are, to be able to articulate her function within them, and then exercise the skills effectively. Usually that comprises the first steps in the role of the managers in the shared governance council. Indeed, they are usually the first council formed in the implementation process.

IMPLEMENTING THE MANAGEMENT COUNCIL

Conceptualizing the management council different from the management committee or team meeting is an important first step. Table 5-1 outlines some of the distinctions of each.

The accountabilities of the management council are directly related to the role of the manager and the power and authority necessary to carry out the defined accountabilities listed above. Accountability determination is therefore one of their first important initial roles. When the SGCC creates and empowers them to begin, the first activity is to delineate as clearly as possible the accountabilities that will initially be necessary for the council to do its work.

When that is done by the management council, the tentative accountabilities are initially approved by the SGCC and can then be implemented by the Management Council (MC). Also, the first chair of the management council is often selected by the SGCC from among its members to ensure consistency between the goals of

FIGURE 5-2
Management council.

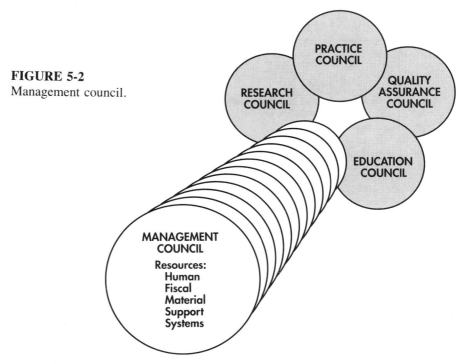

shared governance identified by the SGCC and the role and decisions of the MC.

As shown in Figure 5-2, whatever accountabilities are discerned by this council, they should relate to the functional accountabilities associated with the management role:

Human resources
Fiscal resources
Material resources
Support to staff
Organizational systems

As pointed out earlier, all accountabilities of management should relate to the above role expectations. *The manager is not accountable for the staff roles that relate to practice, quality assurance, education, and research.* Sorting out these accountabilities early helps the shared governance effort by clarifying general accountabilities first so that confusion about where specific roles or obligations belong does not emerge.

The following are some of the initial activities of the management council during its formative period:

Define its reason for being
Outline its purpose and objectives
Select a chairperson
Outline an implementation schedule
Define member tenure, role, expectations, meeting time, and responsibilities
Isolate its accountabilities
Sort out and define the various roles of the managers
Determine the council's level of understanding related to the concept of shared
    governance and its application to management
Establish the powers of the chair
Set the priorities for the year
Construct a manager development plan

TABLE 5-2
Industrial Management Behaviors vs. Shared Governance Management Behaviors

Industrial Behaviors	Shared Governance Behaviors
Directing the staff in their work Approving their ideas or work Seeing to it that the work gets done Granting permission to do things Asking staff for input, then deciding on their behalf Making clinical decisions Rewarding the staff for being "good" (that really means doing what you thought they should do)	Supporting staff in identifying their goals Raising questions important to the staff's work Advising staff with regard to resource implications related to staff decisions Challenging the staff to seek their own solutions Supporting staff in critical decisions and after failure Sharing alternative options in staff planning Assisting in staff problem solving Holding staff accountable for their work Creating an open environment where it is safe for the staff to take a risk and change

The last item on the MC list is a key part of assuring the success of shared governance. In many settings, the failure of shared governance to become what it should relates directly to the inability of the management team to be able to incorporate the essential behaviors into the role of manager. Most of these behaviors relate to the failure to be able to move from the central role of planning, organizing, leading, and controlling for the service she leads to that which facilitates, integrates, and coordinates the staff in doing much of what was once considered part of the manager's role. *Shared governance does not or cannot do away with the role of the manager.* The role, however, has to change dramatically if it is to be effective.

Table 5-2 compares manager behaviors of shared governance and industrial management.

The management council will have to address the behavioral issues outlined in the table in the initial process of implementation. The ability to make these changes will be essential to the successful role of the nurse manager in shared governance. The developmental activities of the MC will therefore have to reflect these changes and represent these developmental issues.

Some suggested topics in the management development process include:

Facilitation vs. direction
Collaborative problem solving
Investing the staff
Group decision making
Equity-based management
Partnering relationships
Coaching skills
Entrepreneuralism and/or intrapreneurialism
Consensus seeking
Meeting management

This list is not exhaustive. The nurse manager will want to add her own items of learning to support her adjustment into a different frame of reference for decision making. Even the openness necessary to make the change results in some positive experiences in the growth of both the manager and the staff.

Management development is so critical that any means necessary to assure it takes place should be sought out. Members of the MC will have their own developmental needs that should be addressed. Indeed, some mechanism should be devised to allow the individual manager to outline her own developmental plan and require her to make progress against some reasonably clear objectives for management effectiveness and behavioral change.

The manager will be the one most responsible for the creation of a safe milieu wherein the staff will begin to take on the issues of their own accountability. Since skills of leadership will be developing in this process, the manager may have to assume the role of model and mentor, as well as stimulator, for the emergence of those behaviors that will strengthen the development of the staff. Since many of these behaviors will be those the manager once was expected to exhibit, the shift will be both a personal journey for the manager and a growth experience for the staff. Clearly some of these efforts will require insight and maturity on the part of the manager.

Some of the behavior adjustments necessary in the role of the manager are as follows:

1. Moving from director to facilitator
2. Altering control to coordination
3. Shifting from managing to integrating
4. Changing focus from unit to system
5. Viewing staff as peers, not subordinates
6. Moving from "Mama" to colleague
7. Teaching problem solving, not problem finding
8. Moving to coaching roles from directing behaviors

The MC must always keep its focus on the resource-related issues that are appropriate to managers. Because of the location and mobility of the manager, she is best able to identify system problems and problems associated with shared governance before staff does (because of their relatively fixed location). In this way the manager can act as problem finder and alert the appropriate leadership individual or forum for appropriate problem solving or solution seeking.

Membership on the management council will vary depending on the shared governance approach and the size of the institution. While most models have all the management team as members of the MC, others, claiming size reduces effectiveness, state that it should be representative just as the clinical councils are. Either approach can succeed. However, the value of full membership in assuring the issues are clear to all sometimes appears to be the system of choice. The need of the organization to have full participation and the ability to deliver a consistent message may have greater weight than the need for a smaller more effective work group. Each setting will have to make those trade-offs based on its own needs and its own culture.

Staff representation is usually an issue of concern also. It is important in shared governance to be able to deliver an appropriate and consistent message. There will be management representation on the staff councils, as we shall soon see. Therefore it is acceptable that there be staff representation on the MC. How much representation depends on the size of the organization and the relationship between the staff councils and the MC. Usually this membership is provided by a staff member who is involved in some leadership role in the shared governance process, either the practice council chairperson or an equivalent. Staff governance leadership is selected because it is believed that there is better connection between the MC and the other governance components and the staff person's credibility on the MC is extended because of the staff member's "official" role in the governance process. The tendency to discount the staff member's role is less of a temptation when he or she has some power to implement change in the organization.

As with all the councils, it is wise to select the chairperson of the MC a year in advance of service and have the person serve as a chair-elect. In this way, the incoming chairperson has a year of council service and the benefit of leadership orientation before filling the role of chairperson. The same skills development and role expectations as identified in the role of the chair of the SGCC apply to the chair of the management council.

In the work of the management council the orientation should always be related to problem solving and outcome achievement. The organization will continue to look to the manager and the management team to exemplify the behaviors and supports that indicate that the movement to shared governance is okay and worth achieving. The role and behavioral changes the manager exhibits reinforce those same expectations of the staff. The staff will be testing, looking, pressing, and questioning the manager's support of this shift in structure and decision making. This council provides the initial impetus for the movement toward shared governance and will become the moderator of the process and its operation. It is a uniquely positioned group to influence and measure the success of the process.

Formation of the council early in the process is a vital step in assuring that the developmental process is not jeopardized. Getting the managers on board early and developing their understanding of the concepts and skills necessary to successful shared governance is a critical element in successful implementation.

The MC must also develop a strong basis for support of the manager, creating a safe place to look for support, identification, problem solving, and emotional support during some of the more challenging change moments. The MC serves as a place for exploring responses to specific problems related to implementation and the need of the manager to know and understand what is happening in the process of implementation. This group serves as a source of clarification and validation in the tentative processes related to implementing the unit-based strategies. Unfolding this is often like writing a script never before devised and living the script as it is written. Needless to say, there will be some rough spots and some places in the developmental process that will be revisited several times. Flexibility and perseverance will be required.

IMPLEMENTING THE PRACTICE COUNCIL

Along with the management council, the practice council is generally a foundation group essential to all shared governance models (see Figure 5-3). It is the primary clinical decision-making group on which all the other groups come to depend. They need the practice council (PC) because of its role in defining the parameters of practice on which the work of the profession builds. Both the work and the leadership of this council are critical to the success of any shared governance model. While it is identified by different names, in a variety of models, its function is always the same: to define and control issues related to clinical practice.

Invested in this council are the powers necessary to make key decisions about clinical practice and the issues that affect it. Often, it is the way the profession defines itself and its boundaries and provides a control mechanism to make sure that ownership gets played out in the organization. As with all other elements of shared governance, decisions made in this group are final and have the power and weight of the profession to support decisions and activities. To use popular euphemisms, it is here where the "rubber hits the road" or the "pedal hits the metal."

The statement of final accountability has historically been okay when applied to the management group; power was always invested in them. It is much more challenging to say that power also rests with others in the organization and then set about certifying that belief by constructing a structure that gives that belief form and direction. This is what the practice council does. It makes the organizational statement that the practicing professional has both the right and a forum for deci-

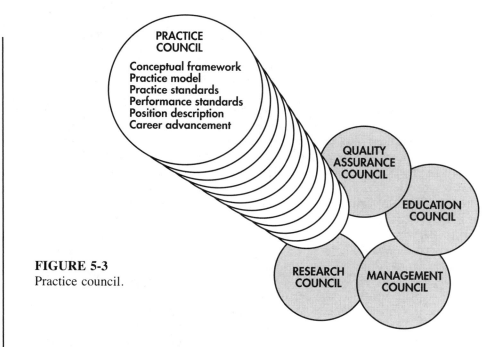

FIGURE 5-3
Practice council.

sion making that affects the work that she does and that authority is equal to the authority that exists in any other place in the organization. Clearly, this is a risky assertion and a major departure from the traditional bureaucratic structuring of authority.

Here the support of the administration is vital to the success of the shared governance model. The reader can see that if that support is missing, the underpinnings of shared governance cannot take hold and the process cannot unfold on firm ground, so to speak. The opportunity to retreat from previous commitments is too easy and sometimes tempting to the administrator, who begins to see the staff actually taking leadership and moving ahead with the process of making meaningful decisions that affect the work they do. The administrative leader is again reminded of these questions:

Do I believe in staff empowerment?

Am I committed to the staff making decisions that affect their work?

Do I trust an organized body of the staff to make good decisions in the best interest of the profession and the workplace?

Will I maintain my support even during trying times?

Do I understand what I am doing?

At the outset, the Shared Governance Coordinating Council usually plays a major role in the selection of the leadership of the PC. The SGCC will want to assure the integrity of the practice council and assure that it fits within the plan for structuring shared governance entrusted to them by the staff. Usually the first chair of this council is selected from the SGCC and plays a major role in the selection of the members of the PC which will be selected from among the staff. Careful consideration of the leadership for this council should be undertaken by the SGCC because of the needs associated with implementing this major decision-making group:

What are the group leadership skills necessary for the chair role?

Can the candidate undertake the group process activities necessary to facilitate discussion?

Does the candidate have a full understanding of the shared governance concept and have the ability to apply it?

Is the candidate a team player?

Are the objectives of implementation of the practice council clear to the candidate?

Does the candidate have the full support of the SGCC?

When the council chair has been selected, membership on the council has to be identified. In the beginning of the shared governance implementation, the method of selection appears to be less important than the kind of person who serves on the council. It appears much more important to have involved and committed individuals involved in the initial stages than it is to see that the staff is broadly represented. This means that, initially, capable people should be identified for membership regardless of where they may come from in the organization.

Although selecting the best staff members may be more important to the implementation process, some organizations have a problem ignoring or depreciating the representational character of membership on the PC. Since that value is fundamental to shared governance, it needs due consideration in planning the first membership. If the SGCC feels that it can obtain the quality of membership and remain appropriately representational, it should do that. The bottom line is this: the best membership that can be obtained at the outset, should be. Remember that representational considerations are fundamental to the developmental process in implementing shared governance. Thus representation issues will emerge early in the process and structures will be devised to assure them. Whether they begin at the point of generating the first clinical council appears not to be as important to the process as having capable and willing members to initiate implementation of the PC.

Membership considerations

Membership on the PC is a more complex consideration than is membership on the management council. Where management council membership is determined by role, membership on the practice council is determined by representation.

Issues related to representation can range from how many members the council should have to where the members should come from. Each institution will have to deal with these issues in a way that reflects its own culture and values. There are some principles that would be helpful to them in making choices. The implementors can check off their own representation process against the following principles:

1. The practice council is a decision-making group. Members should therefore be kept to the lowest possible number. At any rate, the council should have no more than 10 to 14 members. Any size larger than this makes decision making a very difficult process.
2. Staff should always comprise the clear majority of the membership on this council. At least 70% of the members of this group should be selected from among the staff. Other voting members usually include one first line manager, one clinical specialist, and other specialists as defined by the PC.
3. The chair must always be selected from among the staff members. Appointing a manager chair makes the same statement as was always made regarding trust and mistrust in the organization. Staff leadership must be looked at as a viable process and permitted to emerge in legitimate roles. The chair of the practice council is just such a role.
4. Tenure must be established for all members including the chair. Groups with unlimited tenure and the ability to renew membership as an unlimited opportunity creates an elitism that does not encourage staff empowerment or even creativity.
5. A schedule of meetings and meeting times should be published in advance with expectations for attendance. This advance notice should assist in planning for staffing and replacement of members and assure proper attendance at council sessions.
6. Governance sessions are usually considered a part of work-based professional obligations and are therefore paid time. Such meetings are generally scheduled to occur at times when the staff is normally present in the work environment.

The exception will always be the off-shift members who come in at times not considered their scheduled time. These members, too, are paid appropriately for this time.

7. Attendance at governance council sessions generally is considered a commitment. Representatives are usually elected by peers for their roles and represent them in decisions that affect their professional lives and work. They have a right to expect that their representatives are meeting their obligation. The PC should set the required meeting attendance for members and define the consequences of nonattendance up front so that all members are aware of the significance of meeting attendance.

8. The practice council is an authority body that has a defined power to undertake action for which it is accountable. It is not advisory and does not refer its decisions for approval by some other body or person. It is a council precisely because it has authority for its work. Once its accountability has been defined and agreed on, it is free to exercise the authority associated with its accountability. This is what distinguishes shared governance from participatory management systems.

The practice council is uniquely clinical in both design and focus. Here the transformation of the organization is most strongly indicated, and an accountability emerges that exists in no other place in the organization. The staff membership of this council evidences the sharing of power and decision making in ways not expressed in organizations before. It represents the valuation of the profession and the professional and creates the partnership between the professional and the organization. This process exclusively reserves the right of the staff to control their practice and to make decisions that influence both their own practice and the organization.

The practice council cannot know or do its work until the accountability of the council has been clarified and well defined. Dialogue regarding the kind and extent of powers that accrue to the council once its accountabilities are clear becomes important in the effort to certify its role. When those powers are defined, they must clearly reflect the role of the practice council and become inherent in the PC's expression of its role and function in the organization. Here again, it must be emphasized that when accountability has been defined and clarified for this council, it holds those rights and obligations exclusively and must be free to make decisions and to move on them free of constraints not arising from the context of their own deliberations.

The domain of decision making that usually accrues to the practice council includes:

1. The right to define professional practice, including but not limited to the following:
   Conceptual framework
   Philosophy of the profession
   Purposes of the clinical staff
   Critical objectives of the clinical staff
   Relationship of the specific service to other disciplines
2. The obligation to define the role and function of the professional within the context of position descriptions reflecting both the values and conceptual framework of the professional staff.
3. Defining the standards of practice for the profession within the context of the organizational role and culture in providing clinical services. Care standards should also reflect level of accountability and elements of the conceptual framework that describe the profession's value system in the practice setting.
4. Any advancement program that has in part criteria for individual performance that will be measured and thus reflected in the role of the professional.

5. The resolution of interdisciplinary problems that directly relate to clinical practice affecting what workers do or how they do it. Practice-based issues are always the concern and consideration of this council.

Membership selection

As indicated previously, selecting members is a subjective process adaptable to individual settings. The character of the staff mix, service mix, institution size, clinical configuration, medical staff, and so on all serve to influence size and kind of representation on the practice council. Clearly, every member of the staff cannot be a member of the PC. While it is an important group with significant implication for the clinical staff, it must be maintained as a viable decision-making group. This cannot occur if size becomes a constraining issue.

In most settings, selection of members is generally a regional issue. A certain collective of like services join together to select and send the member to make a contribution to the practice council. Usually the member represents the clinical service from which he or she is selected and acts in that role. It is clear that he or she can never adequately represent a service perspective from those units that may be a part of the collective or "cluster," but it must be remembered that when the person is selected, he or she no longer represents any sectional view or issue. The member now becomes accountable for decisions that affect the profession in the institution as a whole and is dealing with all issues from that perspective. That will certainly make the role more challenging with the staff from the areas he or she has been sent; however, the prevailing obligation of the council member is to make decisions in the best interest of the whole rather than the parts at the expense of the whole.

It is important to distinguish between accountabilities that emerge at the unit level and those that fall within the purview of the PC. Most of the issues that will emerge and are of concern to the staff will arise and be resolved at the unit level of the organization. The only concerns that will be addressed by the PC will be issues that affect the profession as a body, result from conflict regarding an issue between two councils, and are related to the profession's goals and objectives as they affect professional practice.

The staff should be aware of the implications of the role and work of the PC. This awareness need not be detailed or even fully understood at the outset. Understanding is a relative condition and often depends on the readiness to hear and the impact of the message on the receiver. Connecting the role of the PC to some value (the work, how the work is done, how much work is done, who does the work, and so on) helps create a reality orientation regarding what is happening in the workplace that is different and how what is happening applies to the individual.

This staff awareness becomes especially important when selection of the representative is occurring. The need to have contributing and thoughtful persons on the PC goes without saying. Finding that person and investing her in the process can at times be challenging. Chances are, however, members on the council will have a variety of backgrounds and abilities to participate fully in deliberations affecting their practice. This reality is not nearly as much of a concern as it may at first appear. Shared governance is a developmental process, and much growth occurs even in the unsuspecting persons. Also, each member brings a set of skills that usually prove to be complementary, and there emerges a broad variety of opportunities to apply them.

Questions are often raised related to educational background needed to undertake a membership role in shared governance, especially on the councils. While it is true the councils, especially the practice council, will be dealing with some complex issues, there is considerable evidence that each level of practitioner has something to contribute to the planning and decision process. The notion that associate degree or diploma education constrains the development and application of shared governance is essentially untrue. The one problem that arises when appraising the contribution potential of, for example, staff nurses, for any given process or event is that their baseline potential is never established. Therefore it is difficult to realize whether there are certain characteristics of shared governance that cannot be addressed by those only basically educated in their discipline. At this stage it appears that the demands of decision making and operating a shared governance approach do not lie outside the behavior or skill parameters of the nurse prepared at the basic level.

What does appear important to the process of shared governance is the preparation of the participant for the role of membership on a governance council. Staff are not prepared to handle as much authority as the councils generate. Often, they are overwhelmed with the activities necessary to make the kinds of decisions arising in the governance format and are somewhat unprepared to undertake governance activities. An orientation to the role of the council member is often helpful in alleviating the concerns that invariably arise; it even generates some new skills helpful in dealing within a deliberative process. Most organizations with shared governance models have some kind of leadership or membership orientation process that includes:

shared governance concepts
problem solving
communication
assertiveness
responsible membership
accountability
representation
council processes and functioning

Armed with these beginning skills, council members have a broader array of skills that can be better applied in the council process and are of benefit in both the practice setting and personal life.

The work of the practice council

The accountabilities of the PC are foundational. Much of the clinical decision making in the service will depend on the outcomes of the PC. The other clinical councils depend on the PC for the foundations on which they will build. The accountability of the PC relates to or builds on the council's work to define and control professional practice. In the shared governance approach, the PC is the place where the exercise of power in relationship to practice emerges and is managed. Because this is true, the delineation of this accountability is essential.

The arena of practice accountability must be clearly articulated by the PC. This serves the purpose of ensuring the work of the PC but also differentiates that work from the work of any other group in the organization (see also Chapter 7 in **Implementing Shared Governance**). If the PC is to be an accountable group, that accountability must not be in evidence in any other part of the institution for those issues over which the PC has designated authority. To do so would negate the effective power of the council to make decisions and to do its work.

The effective powers of the practice council are minimally identified as follows:

Establish the acceptable conceptual base or framework for professional practice

Construct an appropriate definition of care for the practice of the profession

Establish and manage all care standards for the profession or approve those either delegated or emerging from the professional staff

Define and control all clinical job descriptions of the profession including the performance factors or expectations the job description should reflect

Define, control, and manage the career advancement program of the staff

Monitor, alter, and redesign the clinical documentation system for effective recording and evaluation of professional services

These accountabilities form the foundation of the role of the PC. They are not all inclusive but provide the basis on which any shared governance approach can build. Clarity with regard to the PC's role related to these accountabilities is important to formalizing the authority base of the practice council.

It must be remembered that it is not the role of management to define for this group any rules or administrative mandates that might either jeopardize or compromise the authority and/or work of the council. To prevent co-opting the clinical councils, the management role has been kept to a minimum. It is vital that the message that the clinical authority role is comparable to the management role be legitimate and be expressed. Manager members are kept to a minimum. And it is important that the manager representative have a defined role on the council as the representative from the management council or forum so that there is a logical connection between the management process and the clinical decision making.

This separation of authority is not meant to slight or isolate the role of management. Rather, it ensures that there is no confusion or duplication of accountability between those roles that are appropriate to the staff and those that are a part of the manager's obligation. The manager representation provides a linkage between roles and formalizes the governance relationship within the profession between the two key processes essential to the professional work. This linkage is essential to the effective communication and interaction between staff and management. In most shared governance approaches, there is manager membership on all of the staff councils. This ensures that communication between the staff councils and the management council or body is facilitated and that decisional integration is facilitated.

Staff membership on the management council is generally provided in most shared governance approaches. This is an equity-based principle that delivers the message to the nursing organization that representation is a bilateral obligation and represents the best interests of the profession. Usually the representative is drawn from one of the staff councils to ensure the staff representative has some knowledge of the organization and the governance structure and can apply both insight and authority to a role on the management council. Simply selecting the staff member to the management council from the general staff and holding no membership in a formal position of council or governance authority is usually discouraged. Issues related to credibility, power, being sufficiently informed, and so on are often raised when this staff member is not a member of the formal processes associated with shared governance.

More often than not the practice council will be the first focus of conflict in the shared governance approach. Usually, the organization has some issue of reaction that will involve the management and the PC. A conflict in accountability between the management council and the practice council will arise providing the source of the trouble that will test the application of the system. The commitment to dialogue and resolution will be stretched during this set of circumstances. This testing of the system, however, is a necessary adjustment and a possible affirmation of shared governance, if handled appropriately. In the beginning, the SGCC may be the integrating force in the process that can help create a resolution of the difficulty with a positive outcome. The SGCC and the other councils should be

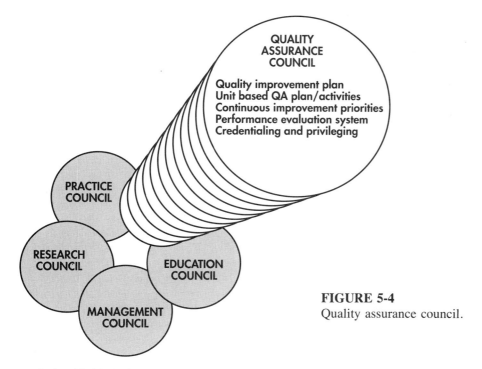

FIGURE 5-4
Quality assurance council.

ready for this kind of challenge to the system. It validates the process and checks the system's ability to deal with present and appropriate conflict. If handled well, it can be indicative of the effectiveness of council-based problem solving.

IMPLEMENTING THE QUALITY ASSURANCE COUNCIL

The second major council group addressed by the SGCC is the Quality Assurance Council (QAC; see Figure 5-4). Some organizations may have already made or be in the process of making the transition from traditional quality assurance approaches to quality improvement. In this book we will use the familiar term "quality assurance" to refer to all quality activities. Readers may substitute the term "quality improvement" for quality assurance to reflect their current approach if they so desire. Whether one adopts a QA or QI philosophy, the implementation process is essentially the same.

The timing of the implementation of the quality council is completely up to the time frame of the SGCC. Sometimes it is wise to wait until the PC is up and running, other times it is good to begin the QAC about the same time as the PC. Usually the councils have much developmental work to do to get their internal operations going. This affects timing insofaras the council's relationship to each other. The QAC depends on the standards development of the PC before it is able to undertake any meaningful work. However, the quality assurance plan must also be in place before the QAC can begin any quality-related activity.

All of the council relationships are subjective and depend on what is in place before their specific work can be clarified. The QAC will always have an interdependent role with the PC and therefore will often depend on PC activities in the course of doing its own work.

The formation of the QAC parallels that of the PC. Both councils are clinically driven and have very much the same staff representation. Again, because it is a clinical council, its chair should also be selected from among members of the staff. The rules for empowering the chair and the roles of the members, tenure, and other considerations very much parallel the work of the PC. Time for its self-work is as important as the other councils and must not be short-circuited so that the council is attending to all the realities that affect its work.

N O T E S

Questions related to membership are slightly different from the PC framework for membership. Some questions include:

What interest do you have in the quality assurance council?

What do you know about quality assurance?

Are you able to take risks in your relationship with your peers?

Can you be firm when standards are at issue?

What does "corrective action" mean to you?

Do you understand that you will be involved in peer-based disciplinary processes?

Have you been personally involved in quality assurance activities?

What makes you want to serve on this council?

Are you willing to give this work a 2-year commitment, if necessary?

Initially the council will focus on its own understanding of the shared governance process and the role quality assurance plays in governance activity. Regarding quality assurance, the following activities will form the core of its initial work:

Understanding current processes associated with shared governance
Reviewing the quality assurance plan
Delineating quality assurance accountabilities and priorities
Establishing the unit-based guidelines and parameters for quality assurance activities
Defining the relationship of career advancement and the evaluation of candidates for advancement
Translating the performance expectations or standards into criteria for performance evaluation
Outlining the elements and processes associated with the credential and privilege process

The quality assurance process often will be the most difficult to undertake in the shared governance approach. It is the governance activity that is most changed and requires the greatest adaptation. From the traditional dislike and mistrust of quality assurance to the dependence on quality assurance as a fundamental part of the operation of the nursing professional activities is a fairly strong leap from historical activity. Most nurses have looked on quality assurance as a necessary evil. In shared governance it becomes a mainstay of professional accountability for which every nurse will have some accountability.

Beside defining the professional basis for relationship and practice, the QAC is the one group that will most often have to connect to other quality assurance activities within the health care setting. All departments and disciplines are required to give evidence of some level of quality assurance activity. In addition, the quality assurance function in each of the services must somehow intersect with others to create an integrative approach to ensure the quality of care. Therefore the QAC must be involved in the following activities:

Agency or institutional quality assurance activities
Interdisciplinary activities that integrate quality assurance activities
Regulatory processes that define the processes the QAC will assess for quality assurance
Defining and exercising activities related to the institution's quality assurance plan
Unit-based quality assurance activities to ensure they are appropriate and consistent with the quality assurance priorities of the organization
Necessary report preparation of its quality assurance activities and its consolidation of those activities with the organization's priorities for quality assurance

Important in the initial work of quality assurance is the definition of the priorities for quality assurance. The clinical units need to have a clear idea of the kind of activities they will be involved in that relate to the priorities for quality assurance for the council. Here the council must give the units some direction with regard to their plan of activities by doing the following:

Defining the framework for quality assurance and outlining quality assurance plan
Establishing the priorities for quality assurance from which the units can develop their plan of QA activities
Delineating the roles in quality assurance that members of the staff must undertake to fulfill their staff requirement for either seeking privileges for practice or applying for employment.
Ensuring the existence of a framework for corrective action that has an impact on every unit's level quality assurance function to ensure compliance with defined expectations

In keeping with the move in health care toward total quality improvement processes, the QAC must be committed to processes that provide for higher levels of function and improvement in the clinical activities of the practitioners. In the past, quality assurance was a process that focused on the quality process as a series of events, which once addressed, were left alone. In shared governance and the continuous quality improvement effort, all quality is an unceasing process that moves along a continuum that in good measure raises the standard and challenges the provider to impart higher levels of practice and care. In this way, quality is a seamless process that does not have a definitive point of achievement; rather, it exemplifies an ongoing series of activities that are continuously altered to reflect higher levels of expectation and performance.

Although implementing the QAC plan is vital to the operation of the clinical organization, it is only one half of the processes associated with the efforts for quality assurance. As indicated earlier, the quality of the care giver is as important as the quality of the care he or she renders. This, too, is a vital part of the quality assurance process.

The board of trustees of the health facility expects that the facility will have on its staff acceptable performers who can fulfill the expectations of their roles. Indeed, it entrusts to the professions the obligation for ensuring that competent staff are available and working in the best interests of the organization and of those it serves. Because the board often cannot judge whether a particular candidate is appropriate for a specific role, it expects that the worker's peers and managers will be able to do that in its best interests and in their own. It is assumed that the profession would not want on staff anyone who would compromise the standards of care that exemplified the values of the profession. While this does not prove true 100% of the time, it is generally accepted that a colleague would not want a worker who is unable to fulfill the expectations of the role or who would violate the standards of the profession.

The quality of the care giver, therefore, is the obligation of the clinical staff. In shared governance this falls within the staff's accountability and authority. Because it is a quality function and builds on the performance standards identified by the Practice Council, the accountability for the mechanism for credentialing and privileging falls to the QAC. Issues that relate to this function follow:

clear definition of the expectations for clinical roles
a mechanism for structuring review of qualifications for clinical positions
a definitive enumeration of the criteria for evaluating credentials
full definition of the accountability of the QAC for evaluation of candidates
an ongoing structure and process for performance evaluation owned by the clinical staff
a context for disciplinary action that is consistent with the privileging process

This mechanism is fundamentally different from any approach to dealing with the staff, especially in relation to competence and shared roles. In shared governance, the peer process takes on important value and the role of the staff is enhanced in the process. The problem is that peer processes have been disparaged in the past. Some of the reasons for this:

No clear criteria that have the confidence of the staff in their fair application of judgment they may make about their peers

A lack of confidence and trust between staff with regard to each other and the ability to objectively relate to the evaluative process

An effective structure for the peer process that uses clear criteria that the individual can control and can be equitably applied to an individual's role

A prevailing belief that evaluation is essentially a punitive or controlling process

The expectation that performance and hiring or firing are specifically management roles for which the staff has only a passive relationship

Clearly, for this process to become an acceptable part of the operation of the professional organization, attitudes and understanding regarding the meaning of the process and its application have to change. The QAC will have to explore all the issues and be fully cognizant of the questions that they will have to face in confronting formation of a peer-based privileging process:

Are the quality assurance criteria specific enough and measurable?

How are the position description elements translated into performance criteria?

How does the peer-based performance evaluation system fit with the career advancement program (career ladder)?

Who is involved in the peer part of the staff evaluation process?

What is the role of the manager in the staff evaluation?

How do performance evaluation criteria fit with the care evaluation process?

What is the mechanism(s) that the QAC will put in place for ongoing performance appraisal?

Is there a critical path for performance evaluation from application for privileges to renewal of privileges in the organization?

How does the QAC assure the board of trustees and administration that the profession's evaluation process is objective and adequate?

This is relatively new territory for nurses and other nonmedical model disciplines. The goal in this process is to access accountability for colleague relationships and provide appropriate competence standards for the profession and the organization within which practice unfolds. Good models for employee-based professional operating systems are just emerging. Therefore much of the work to build good credentialing and peer-based evaluation systems is currently being created. Most organizations will be writing the script as they go.

Some principles will be helpful for the planner in initiating the development of professional credentialing and privileging processes:

1. Consistency in establishing the credential framework for the various services or functions is critical to its being applied equitably to all candidates for positions.
2. Definitive standards for acceptable certifications must be developed. As much as possible, national or discipline defined standards or certification requirements should always take precedence.
3. Generic credentialing standards should always be developed first and used as the basis for service and institution-specific credentials requirements in order to establish a premise for consistency.
4. The QAC should have a mechanism that establishes the role of each group or individual in the credentialing process that can operate without the direct intervention of the QAC in the ongoing program.
5. Most of the credentialing and privileging process should occur at the unit level. Peer relations and accountability should provide the foundation for the program, this always occurring at the practice level.
6. Credentialing for management and practice candidates should be a separate process with activities designed in each for the role of the other in the credentialing process.
7. The credentialing and privileging process for staff should be staff driven with the final approval of candidates for practice privileges resting with the QAC.
8. The right to credential and privilege is a Board of Trustee prerogative delegated to the profession acting on behalf of the board. Board approval and acceptance of the credentialing and privileging process *must* occur at some time in the implementation process before it can be an official or acceptable operating process.
9. Managers *always* play a role in credentialing and privileging because of their resource accountability. That role is most often included in the unit process.
10. The bylaws must spell out the credentialing and privileging process of the professional service in understandable and applicable terms. This ensures that a consistent and replicable process is in place and can be applied in any setting.

Needless to say, credentialing processes are not the first agenda item for the QAC. There is much preparatory work before this process is in place. It depends on several organizational factors operating in the clinical system:

A conceptual model has been selected.
Clinical standards of practice are present.

Performance standards have been developed and form a basis for evaluation processes.

A staff-based performance evaluation system is operating.

The quality assurance program is running effectively.

Goals and objectives and council priorities have been constructed and are in place.

The QAC, along with its work, is not initially one of the easiest groups with which to interest the staff. In addition to appearing hard to understand, a great deal of work seems attached to the quality improvement process. While this insight is true, the council also has the most profound impact on the staff and influences who can be a member of the staff and what staff do in their professional roles in the organization. In time, it is one of the more sought after groups in the shared governance process.

IMPLEMENTING THE EDUCATION COUNCIL

The Education Council (EC) is primarily responsible for issues related to professional competence (see Figure 5-5). Factors associated with maintaining ongoing competence and continuing education are also the main focus of this group. The change in the organization recognizes that the staff has a strong obligation for the continuing and ongoing competence of its members. That obligation is a collateral accountability in that each member of the staff has the obligation to be competent in his or her practice and ensure that all others are as competent. The issue in a professional framework is that those who do the work of the profession must be mutually able to do it and maintain the requisites during the extent of their tenure.

Again, this council is a clinical council and has the same membership characteristics as the Practice Council. Because of the unit-based focus of a great deal of shared governance education processes, there are often more members from the staff on this council than on the other clinical councils because each unit is represented. There is no structural reason why this must be so; however, specific settings have program structures that call for unit representation. As can be assumed, if implementation were taking place in a large organization, it could create a great

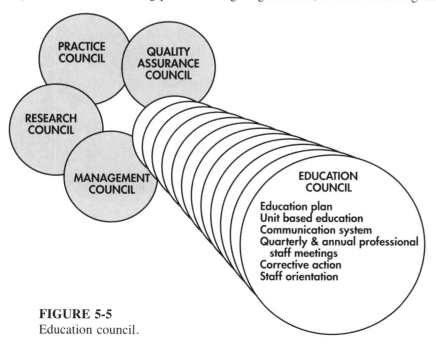

FIGURE 5-5
Education council.

N   O   T   E   S

deal of difficulty in both organization and cost to have such a large council. Here again the tension is between effectiveness and size as it is with all the councils. Because of the wide diversity of functions the tendency for all the councils is to enlarge rather than keep the groups to a manageable size; however, a membership of 7 to 10 is best.

Historically, it has been considered the obligation of the institution to ensure that its *employee* is competent. There has been no belief that the professional worker brings that obligation with him or her and that activities related to ensuring competence remain within the context of that individual's responsibility. The employee relationship changed the locus of control for this issue and illegitimately placed it into the institutional hands. Since that process is in place, all regulators and accreditors now expect the institution to manage staff education.

Clearly the introduction of accountability-based approaches challenges some of the prevailing operational beliefs. The following questions help to focus the issue more clearly:

Where is the nursing education located on the organizational chart?

What does the nursing education department (or hospital education department) do regarding professional education?

What is the role of the individual professional in managing his or her own education program?

Do staff teach each other in the formal education program as a primary professional obligation?

Is education unit or department based rather than centralized?

Is all professional education patient focused, and, at times, does it include the patient?

Who keeps the staff member's education record, the staff member or the institution?

Does the staff member use the education record as a performance validation tool in his or her performance evaluation?

The obligation of the staff member for his or her own education has been an expectation of the profession but not structured into the organizational system where nurses practice. In shared governance, the whole process of competence delineation moves to the accountability of the staff. Structures are provided that ensure that education- and competence-based activities are incorporated into the obligations of each staff member.

Included in the consideration of the EC's work is the development of both standards and processes for the transition of this process from the organization to the EC. It is not the obligation of the EC in shared governance to do all the activities now associated with the education department. The accountability, however, does transfer to the EC. In effect, the education service or department is accountable to the professional body for its activity. In this professional model, the EC defines the expectation, roles, and services provided it by the education service. Of course, in most organizations with shared governance, the education department leadership has representation on the EC. Here again, the staff election and representation process models what has occurred in the other clinical councils. The development of operating rules and regulations and the issues of service and tenure parallel what has happened in the other councils. Since this is a staff council, it is assumed, as with the other clinical councils, that the majority of members are from among the practicing staff.

Communication

While the traditional issues that affect staff competence are certainly a part of the role of the EC, the whole arena of effective communication in the shared governance system is also a major consideration for the EC. Since education is primarily a process of communication, the connection of the communication system with the EC is both logical and appropriate. In most shared governance models the EC is generally responsible for constructing and managing the professional communication model. Some of the elements addressed in developing this accountability are identified below:

Generating information among the councils for their connectedness and effective problem solving

Producing data related to shared governance activities for the organization's leadership or for specified purposes

Informing the staff regarding the activities of the leadership and the activities of shared governance

Communicating between the councils and the staff as a whole at a regular interval for staff feedback and input on the activities of the councils

Creating an annual process that reviews the goals and objectives of the organization, selects the staff leadership, reports on council outcomes, and celebrates the staff accomplishments

Generating a staff newsletter or other communication device where the staff can communicate their own impressions, issues, professional values, research, and other matters of concern to the staff and the councils

There is often much discussion about the development of peer relations in the professions. The format for peer processes is often not present in the organization, making it difficult for the staff to really identify what kinds of relationships they want and how to develop them. The staff always note that there is little enough time to devote to establishing ways of communicating and relating to each other in a more formalized way. At the same time, they admit that such relationships are essential to good working relationships. The EC makes such issues its concern, and the possible mechanisms for peer interaction and process are explored with the outcome, an organized way of accomplishing these relationships. Such processes as those that follow are often considered.

Unit-based staff meetings that include staff roles in reporting, problem solving, and even socializing

Informal and social opportunities for staff to get together to meet, discuss issues of common concern, or simply to build community

Continued education offerings created by the staff for themselves and/or connecting to other professionals in the community or outside of their own service frame of reference

Informal or formal meetings with other disciplines for dialogue and problem solving and, as appropriate, socialization

Clearly the work of the EC is important to the milieu of the professional organization. It can often set the framework for shared governance growth and development. A focus on the context and the behaviors associated with professional activity helps maintain the structure or context of shared governance and provides a vehicle for educating the staff and keeping them invested from within the organizational system.

Important, too, are the orientation processes associated with shared governance. The entire orientation program falls within the auspices of the EC. Here again, it is important that the context for shared governance be communicated to the future member of the staff as soon as possible. A new professional is orienting not only to the work but also to the relations that make up the work place. The EC has a major responsibility to see to it that the candidate has the opportunity, the tools, and the expectation to both perform and behave in a way that empowers, enables, and interacts well with peers and their governance processes. Therefore the orientation process should contain at least the following elements as it relates to shared governance:

The structure of the shared governance format

The role of the staff in a shared governance structure

The obligations of staff members for practice, quality, and competence in shared governance processes

The election or selection processes associated with representation on the governance bodies

The role of the staff on career advancement (ladder) programs and the governance-related activity for advancement

A basic review and beginning understanding of the rules, regulations, and bylaws that govern the activities of the professional staff and the individual's role in governance.

The Education Council sets the context for shared governance in its strong focus on the professional issues that directly affect what the staff do, essentially, for themselves. Some have said that the EC focuses on the person of the nurse rather than the process of nursing (or any practice). This council personalizes the activities of shared governance and often serves to make them real for the individual. It puts a human face to shared governance because it works to connect staff to each other in both formal and informal ways. Through its strong role in communication and managing the communication system, the EC maintains the close connection to and between the staff. Since it is communication based, it serves to maintain the focus of that role as an ongoing part of its activities.

Relationship to other councils

The EC is most dependent on and directly related to the other clinical councils. Often education work of the EC reflects what has been done by the other councils. To the extent the other councils generate new standards, practices, or processes associated with changing practice or staff behavior, the practice council becomes important to the educational and developmental needs of the staff. The other clinical councils become dependent on the organizational-educational role of the EC for the implementation of education related to major change.

Here again, a level of tension exists between the legitimate educational work of the EC and that of the other councils. The EC is not to become simply a vehicle for the other councils to do their work with the staff. As with all change, there is an educational role related to the activities of each council. It should not be anticipated that the other councils conceive and then direct the education council to develop the staff to do as the other councils direct. There is an equity of accountability between the councils, and the EC has defined roles and functions as identified above, just as the other councils do.

Each council must take on that component of program development or change that addresses its own concerns. When that requires an education component, they may look to the EC for assistance in planning and structuring but the work of processing education associated with the undertaking belongs to the originating council. Education will always be part of the work of the councils. In this case, education falls within the context of the work of the program or the initiative of the generating council.

Still, the EC will depend a great deal on the work of the other councils, especially the practice and the quality assurance councils, since much of the formative and structural work will be done by them. From those practice- and quality-based structures much of the education process will take form and will be the basis of some of the work of the EC.

Usually the EC begins somewhat after the time that management, practice, and quality assurance activities get generated in the organization. Because it depends on some of the practice and clinical processes being clearly structured and articulated, the EC will usually be initiated about 6 months to 1 year after the other two councils are formed. This gives them time to do their initial work and to provide a framework with which the EC will build its activities.

Although beginning the EC later than the Practice and Quality Assurance councils is the general approach to implementation, it is not essential. There are many organizations whose sophistication of activities is such that the essential undertaking of the practice and quality assurance processes is sufficient to get the EC going and have it pursue some of its own developmental work. It must be remembered by the implementors that the "self-work" of each council is such that it takes about 3 to 4 months to get the operating mechanics worked out so that it can effectively begin its work with all the functional capabilities of a governance group.

IMPLEMENTING THE RESEARCH COUNCIL

In keeping with the five delineators of a professional group (practice, quality, competence, research, management), it is important that research be incorporated into the implementation discussion (see Figure 5-6). It is clear that not all service settings will be adequately prepared to discuss the development of the research governance component and may therefore select to leave this process until much later in the developmental process. Indeed, many shared governance organiza-

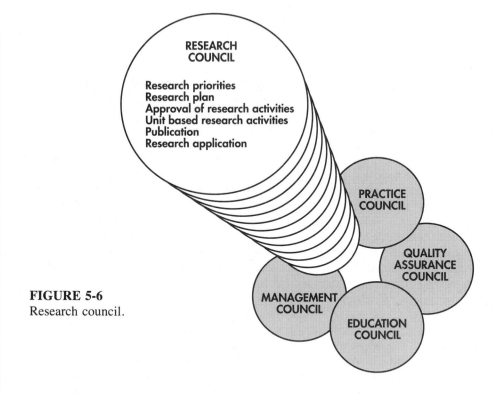

FIGURE 5-6
Research council.

tions, otherwise operating very effectively, have not addressed the professional accountability related to the research process.

Several issues affect consideration of the implementation of the research accountability within the shared governance format:

> There is an organized research activity within the organization.

> A research office (planned?) coordinates the discipline's research activity.

> Sufficient resources are committed to the research activity to support research projects.

> Staff are involved in and value research activities.

> Research activities result in some practice impact in the organization through an organized system of implementation.

Most nursing and other professional organizations do not have a formalized or highly developed research function. Therefore there is usually much preliminary work to do to formally express the professional accountability for research. Planning activities related to setting up the Research Council (RC) could be some of the first activity of the council group if there is sufficient evidence of organizational support for the clinical research process. Because of the newness of the research approach in most clinical departments, the activities of research and preparation for them usually must begin in a very early planning format. Questions related to the possibilities of a governance structure for research might be these:

Is there sufficient evidence of support for research by the clinical staff?

Identify three reasons why it appears that research activities can begin:

   1.

   2.

   3.

Where is the leadership for this activity coming from—management or staff?

Are staff-driven practice, quality, and competence structures (practice, quality assurance, and education) progressing well at the unit level?

Does nursing (or clinical service) have a relationship or membership on the Institutional Review Committee?

Are there clearly identified leadership persons willing to facilitate the development of the research function through all the phases of implementation?

Because organized research activities are rarely found in most service settings in the United States, it will be difficult to move the process along without some challenge. Aside from the organizational challenges, most practitioners will have some difficulty "buying into" the process of research. Many will see it as an additional activity; others will remember that it was a difficult process to comprehend in their academic experience and will be reticent to consider research a part of their professional role. Implementors will have to anticipate these realities as they plan for this governance function.

The initial interest and developmental activities will have to answer the following questions:

N   O   T   E   S

What is the level of staff understanding about the research process?

What information is available to facilitate an understanding of research in the staff?

What is the value of clinical research in the organization?

What research is currently done in the organization? Who is permitted to do it?

What material and other informational resources are available to expand staff understanding of the research process?

Developmental activities for the research council

The process of moving to a governance structure for the research function will take a considerable period of time. The following steps and processes will have to be included in any effort to implement the RC:

Format the RC as a beginning group designated to do some of the formative work in preparation for the council format.

Outline the council's philosophy, purpose, and implementation objectives.

As with the other councils, format the operating rules and regulations within which the council will operate.

Develop a basic research activities plan that focuses on the research elements and processes of the council.

Accelerate the developmental level and understanding of the council members regarding the research process.

Develop the research application and approval process.

Establish the criteria for external participation in research activities.

Establish the research priorities for the clinical service.

Define the unit-based connection to the research process and the RC.

Define the authority relationship between the RC and the Institutional Review Committee.

Define the university and/or academic relationship (if any) established within the auspices and control of the RC.

Identify the resource-related processes of funding, paying for, and supporting research activities.

Disseminate research findings to staff and other leadership in the organization.

Establish the nursing role and participation in the institutional product evaluation process.

Undertake evaluation studies of operational and structural processes affecting the appropriate delivery of nursing services.

Obtain the literature and funding source information as a part of the effort to make the research process self-supporting.

Design and complete a developmental plan for the RC that would include at least the following:

Research priorities

Accountability (autonomy, authority, and control)

Piloting (if appropriate)

Administration (or staff functions)

Essential relationships

Financing plan

Reporting-publishing activities

The activities of the RC will necessitate the clinical staff being involved to a greater extent in research activities than has been previously expected in most health care organizations. To do so will require careful consideration and planning. Whatever research activities will be undertaken, they cannot appear to add to the workload of the staff. Whatever is initiated by the RC will have to fit within the existing workload arrangements of the staff and will therefore require the establishment of a close working relationship with the practice, quality assurance, and education councils. Data collection activities, as well as research design processes, will have to be incorporated into both clinical care and documentation processes already in place. Included in the strategy of implementation should be the following elements:

A method for systematically identifying patient care problems (usually quality assurance)

A clearly defined research format

A mechanism for incorporating research designs

Formats or document design supportive of research

A mechanism for changing research-generated practice activities

Organized mechanisms for disseminating research data or outcomes

A way to manage research-based funds

An organizational standard or policy requirement for participation in research activities (sometimes included in the career advancement program)

The planning for the formation of the research council should occur in the initial stages of the planning for shared governance. It may not be realistic for the council to take form until the staff is far along in the developmental process. The work of the other councils becomes important, indeed, takes priority because of their foundational work. Often, many of the processes needed by the research council will be developed by one of the other councils. The work of each developed council should assist the efforts of subsequent councils. *There is no need to reinvent the wheel: preparation by one council in relation to structure and organization should be replicated by the subsequent councils in their own development, to the extent applicable.* Because so much of the work of the RC is developmental, it has the potential to benefit most directly from the work already accomplished by the other councils, especially the quality assurance council. Good communication among the councils from the outset is essential to the success of the process.

THE ROLE OF THE EXECUTIVE COUNCIL

As indicated in the previous sentence, communication is essential to the success and facilitation of the implementation of shared governance activities. Initially the Shared Governance Coordinating Council plays that role. It provides the base for development and communication of all the activities in implementing shared governance. It moderates and monitors the implementation activities and deals with the problems and issues associated with unfolding the shared governance concepts. Integration of the developmental processes is central to the activities of the coordinating council.

The tenure of the SGCC is directly related to the implementation of the governance councils (practice, quality assurance, education, research, and management). As the councils operate more independently with anticipated outcomes, the value of the SGCC begins to diminish. Since its function is directly related to the implementation process, its value in the governance integration function is relatively minor. However, integration becomes vitally important in the governance activities as the councils produce more outcomes and begin to have an impact on the functional activities of the organization. As this occurs, the SGCC becomes less effective or appropriate and must consider ending its work and making the transition to the development of the Executive Council (see Figure 5-7). This usually begins to become evident after the first year following the full implementation of the practice, quality assurance, education, and management councils. It is not a sudden revelation but a transitional process where the need and effectiveness of the SGCC begin to diminish.

The transition to the executive council

Originally the SGCC was broadly constructed with a great number of categories of professional representatives. This strong and diverse grouping from the discipline ensured that initial structures and processes associated with shared governance had extensive dialogue and ample support. As the structures take form and the councils do the work for which they were empowered, the design issues take on less significance and integration issues become paramount. Since this issue relates to governance integration, a structural adjustment or shift will be necessary.

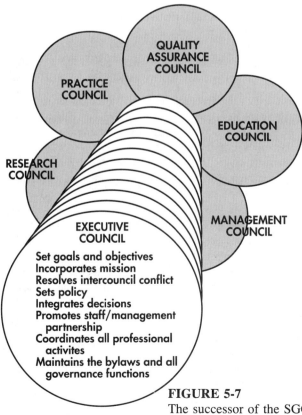

FIGURE 5-7
The successor of the SGCC: the executive council.

This shift can be facilitated if planned for at the outset of the formative processes of the SGCC. As indicated at the outset in the discussion of the SGCC's work, one of the main functions of the SGCC is to work itself out of operation as the other governance functions began to accomplish what is expected of them. A transitional time frame can be used as a way of evaluating the appropriate time and mechanism for making the change.

Questions asked to indicate the time for change may include the following:

Are all the anticipated council formats currently implemented?

Are the issues being addressed by the SGCC of a structural or functional nature?

Has it been a year to a year and a half since the SGCC was formed?

Yes (Should be close to closure) No (Problems?)
       Work left to be done:
       1.

       2.

       3.

       4.

       5.

Council chairpersons are in place and operating effectively?

Councils are on course in undertaking their work?

More work is unfolding in the councils rather than the coordinating council?

The answers to these questions should provide the information that will help the SGCC decide its own readiness and timing of change. It should be remembered that the process of bringing closure to the group will be difficult. A group has a life of its own. Relationships are established, bonds are formed, and positive and creative outcomes are achieved. The group becomes an extension of its members. They are reluctant to disband and often can find many reasons to continue.

The expressive power of this group is extensive. When the SGCC brings closure to its work, the impact of the shift of power becomes clear. Here again, it is often difficult to actually give over that power to the emerging leadership. The ownership and investment of the SGCC members are powerful and can really prohibit or slow the transfer of the power. A plan of transition can be very helpful in this regard, giving the transition some parameters. The following can help in the transitional process:

A timetable for transition
An evaluation tool to assess readiness
Completion of predetermined activities
Subsequent activities for group members
A mechanism for personal transitioning
A way of acknowledging accomplishments
A social or symbolic activity of transition

Perhaps the most effective way of facilitating the transition to the executive council is to incorporate the formation of the ExC in the transition of the SGCC. Many facilities have the charter (first) chairpersons of the individual councils selected from the SGCC or, if not, they become members of the SGCC on their initial selection. In this way a tie exists between each of the governance councils and the SGCC at the outset. At a predetermined time members, not council chairpersons, transition off the SGCC and are not replaced. This usually occurs over the first 1 to 2 years of implementation so that at the end of the second year only the council chairpersons remain members of the SGCC and they can then make the transition more easily into the ExC.

The ExC is the integrating group made up of the elected chairpersons of the governance councils and the chief nursing (or service) officer of the department, division, or service. This council focuses entirely on the role of integration. It has no accountability of its own, since only the governance councils can express professional accountability as can the chief nursing (or service) officer. The ExC is delegated responsibility by the councils and the administrative leadership for integrating the activities of governance and the operation of the organization. It is the place in the service where the partnership (remember, shared governance is a partnership between the profession and the organization) gets played out. It is where the profession and the organization come together to fulfill the mandates or requisites of their relationship. The following activities are most noted as the work of this body:

Problem solve between and among the governance councils.

Settle disputes between the councils regarding issues of accountability.

Formulate the goals and objectives of the organization.

Merge the mission, purposes, and goals of the organization with those of the profession.

Evaluate the effectiveness of the shared governance structures.

Approve the budget and other policy or process functions of the service as a whole.

Remove chairpersons not functioning appropriately for their role or obligation.

Construct and control the bylaws.

Report shared governance activities regularly to the staff.

Represent the profession and organization at formal processes as indicated.

Those who worry that this body may be the implementation of another hierarchical function must remember that its only obligation is to integrate the organization. None of the accountabilities of the councils can be taken on by this group. It cannot assume accountabilities that belong to the councils. Its first obligation is to see that difficulties in function and accountability can be resolved by the appropriate councils. When that is not possible, then it does have the right to resolve the difficulty. First, it assigns resolution to the council it deems to be the appropriate one. If this fails, only then can it actually act to define the solution to the issue.

The ExC acts more as a court of last resort than a source of directing activity in shared governance. The directing function must rest with the governance councils, which are the only legitimate authorities for such activity. The ExC is a trust extended by the staff and the councils to ensure that linkage between the councils, staff, management, and board is in place and that the desired and designed system of shared governance operates as structured. The ExC must ensure that it continues to operate in the best interest of the organization and the profession whose partnership it represents.

The nurse executive (or service executive) is a member of this group and provides the following role and activities within the group:

Links the ExC with the board and administrative goals, plans, and processes influencing the operation of the service

Provides information essential to executive decision making and planning and access to other information resources affecting quality decisions

Serves as a forum for the visions, plans, and notions of the executive regarding the effective functioning of the service and the merging of mission and purposes of the organization with those of the profession or service

Processes issues of conflict between the organization and the profession directed to solution seeking

Serves as a safe place for dialogue with regard to the constraints of the organization and the strategic activities to address the challenges of the organization in meeting its service objectives

Leads the evaluation of the effectiveness of the shared governance system and proposes adjustments and enhancements to more effectively accomplish the work of the profession and the organization.

The issue of the executive's role in a shared governance approach is always in question. It becomes an emotional issue when all the personal and power ramifications are included in the discussion. The issue of veto is always lingering in the wings on the stage of the discussion regarding the authority of the executive in shared governance.

Shared governance as a concept does not value the notion of veto. If the shared governance structure is formatted appropriately and effectively, the decisions that would historically require a veto are made in a way that a veto process would be a moot consideration. The executive's use of a veto is virtually always a sign that the appropriate decisional processes, so much a part of shared governance, were not appropriately used, were bypassed, or were poorly organized. Use of veto is more a sign of a collapse in the structure of shared governance or of the executive's lowered level of trust in the system's ability to effectively do what it is constructed to do. Either way, its use is indicative of failure in the system, not effectiveness or efficiency, as is often claimed.

The ExC should serve as a forum for those issues that, in other circumstances, would be dealt with only by the upper management leadership in the service. It is important to recognize that confidential and important issues to the service and the discipline can be as effectively discussed and dealt with in the ExC as any decisional group. An old adage is, that given the same information, the same skills, the same opportunity, the same time, people will generally make the same decision. Decision making has less to do with who makes decisions than the resources available to assist persons in making sound decisions. It should be the intent, indeed, the goal of the executive to see that access to whatever the ExC needs to facilitate effectiveness in its work is always available and can be provided to this leadership group in the same way it might be provided to the management team.

The notion of "stakeholding" becomes important in the shared governance concept and the role of the ExC. It is a fundamental belief of the whole approach that all professionals have some ownership over what they do in the context of their discipline. Because of this and because of what they have invested in the organization, and what staff has done to fulfill its goal, a partnership exists between the profession and the organization with both parties to the relationship having a shared outcome resulting from their interaction.

It is this concept of partnering that is most represented by the ExC. The selected leadership and the executive leadership join in this council to deliberate in the best interests of both to best fulfill the mission and purposes of the health care entity including all those issues that might affect the relationship itself. Since all will benefit by the work of this group, it best exemplifies the mutuality expressed in the shared governance structure.

The implementor should not, however, assume that all goes well and that a short cut to heaven has been obtained through the shared governance route. Clearly, in an imperfect world, many issues will demand continued effort. There will never be a time when absolute consensus will be achieved. There will always be those who do not agree that the best possible outcomes have been achieved. There will also be those times when the decision made at one time will have to be later adjusted because the information available is better or leads to different conclusions. These and other variables will always serve to keep the tension of circumstances and issues influencing the process and the outcome. Openness to the process and commitment to the approach of shared governance will be necessary; if present, these will, in the long run, positively support the most appropriate consequence.

In building the long-term effectiveness of the ExC the leadership will be confronted with issues from a number of forums. Some of the issues that emerge along the way are:

The role of the medical staff leadership who seek to have a voice in decisions that affect their practice

The selection of a chairperson or president of the nursing staff. Who should that be? What role will he or she play? What is the relationship to the executive? To the staff? How will the person be selected?

The relationship between the profession within the organization and the professional bodies outside the workplace

Nursing staff leadership emerging in the political or community arenas and the impact on the organizations within which they practice

Critical problem solving between nurses and administrative leadership when the crisis relates to direction, resource allocation, and economic issues

Impact of shared governance as an operating process within the larger workplace arena, especially in changing the characteristics of employment law, labor relations, and the accreditation processes

These and other issues will always confront the leadership as the behaviors supporting professional action begin to take form. As the whole shared governance organization begins to have an impact on the organization beyond the issues of the discipline, the ExC must be willing to integrate those issues and structures into the dialogue and into changing the format of shared governance and the relationship of the discipline with other components of the organization and institution of which nurses and other professionals are a part.

Shared governance as a concept or process is not the property of any one discipline. It is a vehicle for operation and for change. It can work for any and all disciplines. The model used in this workbook is specifically directed to the professional worker and organization and defines structure within that format. It can be modified to almost any work circumstance that involves a preponderance of knowledge workers. It is a less effective model for exclusively vocational or technical workers or those whose learning or work is based essentially in an on-the-job training or learning model.

For those who are interested in incorporating the technical, clerical, or assistive personnel in the decision-making format of shared governance there are a number of options the ExC may use to make that decision.

The nonprofessional groups may select one member for one or the other practice council depending on the focus of their work (e.g., management council for the clerical worker or practice council for the clinical assistants).

Council members may be assigned to any one of the technical, clerical, or assistive personnel committees or work groups and act as their liaison to the governance council(s). Representation would come from a council most aligned with the committee or work group seeking a connection to the council(s).

No connection between the technical, clerical, or assistive workers is made at the divisional council level. Representation is expected at the unit level where these workers are scheduled and where they have their voice.

A body made up of all nonprofessional workers meets with the representative from the ExC and the executive to deliberate issues of concern to them. Their members are selected by their co-workers and have a regular agenda and scheduled function within the organization that connects to the ExC rather than to the governance council(s).

N   O   T   E   S

All these issues affecting the professional workplace as a whole that are not a part of the appropriate individual accountability of the governance councils fall within the context of the ExC. The goal of this group is to see that the system functions equitably and effectively and that brokenness anywhere in the process is addressed and the shared governance operation is consistent and contiguous.

Unit-Based Shared Governance Activities

Shared governance really does not take form until it is present in the places where the staff does its work. Unit-based activities in shared governance are important components of the shared governance process (see Chapter 4 in **Implementing Shared Governance**). Either the division-wide or department-wide approaches are essential for the shared governance process to be complete. The checks and balances necessary to ensure a balance between the two are important structural parameters. They ensure that each forum is not doing the work of the other and that expectations for the unit are not the same as those for the governance (divisional or departmental) councils.

All of the behaviors of shared governance actually emerge in the units or workplaces where the staff spend their clinical lives. All of the changes in shared governance should be directed to that end. Actual change in the approach emerges in the units. While there is certainly change in the council membership, broad-based changes in the staff occur in the work setting.

STRUCTURE

There is a lot of discussion regarding just how unit-based models should "look." Because of traditional thinking about organizational consistency, there is some feeling that unit models should match or reflect the governance councils. As most people are aware, each organizational system or work unit is designed ostensibly to respond to the service demand and work culture of the unit. Every unit of service is different from every other unit. There is no service consistency, nor should there be. If clinical departments are to be constructed to provide appropriate service within the context of demand and nature of service, they will necessarily reflect a unique set of organizational characteristics. Replicating the divisional or departmental governance model universally on multiservice, multilateral unit services would be inappropriate and ineffective. It is better to allow the units to create their own internal structures. The caveat to this should be the requirement that every work unit apply the prevailing principles of shared governance as articulated by the ExC to their own unit development. These principles can act as an overlay (template) to the units' shared governance efforts to validate their implementation strategies. This allows for consistency in principle and diversity in design.

READINESS

All work units will reflect a different level of readiness for implementation. A number of factors influence this:

The knowledge of the unit with regard to the shared governance concept

The unit manager's understanding and readiness for the changes the shared governance approach may indicate

The nature and kind of staff that make up the unit from high per diem to long-term staff have a different impact on implementation

The degree of participation already present on the unit as facilitated by the nurse manager

The interest in the staff for maturity or adult relationships and behaviors

The service administrator's ability and willingness to risk the degree of change that will occur at the unit level

The ability of the system to allow the "noise" of change to occur with all the risks inherent in that process

The rate at which change is generally acceptable in the setting and the willingness to initiate the process in order to get things started

The willingness of staff and management to confront the fear of honesty, of directness, and of the more uncomfortable issues that will invariably emerge.

There is no such thing as readiness for change. People are rarely ready for change—change simply happens! Waiting for readiness simply means waiting. It usually indicates that the comfort level, information level, or risk level is not sufficient for undertaking the commitment that such a change requires. Focus on readiness most often means focus on fear. All of the above characteristics will never be sufficiently ready to implement change. The timing of change depends on many factors, the least of which is readiness. Choice of a change is strategic and depends on how much preparation, consideration, and willingness to risk have been anticipated and incorporated into the planning process. The model and format for the change are the vital elements that give any change process some structure. If well conceived and well planned, the degree of risk is reduced and the chances of success are accelerated. Readiness has very little to do with it.

Questions regarding the preparedness of individual units must be raised and answered by both staff and management:

What are the three most important factors inhibiting change to unit-shared governance?

     1.

     2.

     3.

What are three factors that facilitate changing now to a shared governance format?

     1.

2.

3.

Questions for the nurse manager:
What do I know about shared governance?

Is it enough? Do I need more? What do I need?

How do I feel about shared accountability?

What have I done to "free" my staff?
1.

2.

3.

4.

5.

Do I believe in collateral accountability (staff having equal authority, autonomy)?

Do I feel willing to risk a major change in this unit and staff at this time?

Have I reviewed all available literature on unit-based shared governance?

Do I have a notion of the event, crisis, or situation that will serve as a catalyst for getting started?

The following opportunities exist as a format for starting shared governance activities:

Self-scheduling

Standards development

Practice model changes

Work redesign

Unit location move

Change of manager

New unit

Other:_____
_____
_____
_____

Is administration supportive of the move to shared governance?

Does this unit have good communication and relationship with the other units implementing shared governance in order to discuss opportunity and problems?

Unit size will often affect the degree of preparedness and the kind of model that will be selected or created by the individual unit. Smaller units may have one staff council that deals with all the clinical accountability and issues of the unit including those related to practice, quality assurance, education, and research. Other larger units will have all the above issues addressed in the appropriate unit councils. Other units may have a different set of forums or groups for expressing staff accountability. The requirement is the staff expression and formalization of their accountability. If they can give the governance councils evidence of such shared accountability, there should be no issue with regard to the "how" they have chosen.

A great deal of flexibility should be given to the units as they struggle with the most appropriate format for their shared governance activities. As much resource support should be available to them as possible in the process. There must be incorporation of the governance representative framework in the unit design so that there can be appropriate council connection at the unit level. If the individual governance councils have a difficult time determining their accountability relationship to each unit, it will be problematic for the system in determining whether its authority has connected with the unit and that the obligations for performance have been acted on by the unit staff.

The concept of clustering is used often to address this relationship between unit and governance councils. This concept creates a group of representatives from similar or like units (e.g., medical, critical care, specialty, and so on). This group meets to discuss issues of mutual concern or to problem solve or even support implementation activities. They also connect directly to the governance councils for referring issues or implementing decisions of the governance council(s). In some settings, the cluster selects their representatives to the governance councils. Those members connect the cluster directly to the larger governance bodies providing the direct linkage between the unit staff leadership and the councils, thus integrating all levels of the organization. The clusters then assume some authority for assuring the units' compliance with expectations or obligations. Also, this process strengthens the problem-solving process related to issues of conflict or concern. Again, this clustering notion depends on the kind of governance model chosen, the size of the hospital, and the connection between unit and governance bodies. Clearly, the smaller hospital would have unit representation to the councils where the larger institution would be precluded by size to accomplish the same kind of representation.

Units need to raise questions regarding their specific relationship to the governance councils by indicating how the various council accountabilities are to be manifested on their individual units:

What is the mechanism for staff ownership in making practice decisions on the unit?

       Standards development

       Job descriptions

       Career ladder (clinical)

       Performance standards

       Clinical problems

       Interdisciplinary concerns

       Format for problem solving

       Linkage to the Practice Council

How does staff ensure the connection of the unit to the assurance of quality nursing care?

      Application of the quality assurance plan

      Individual staff QA activities

      Peer process in QA

      Peer evaluation plan and process

      Credentialing and privileging

      Corrective measures and actions

Is the education requirement connected to the staff in a way that it can be met in the practice arena?

      Unit education plan

      Individual education plan

      Patient-based education program

      Unit orientation plan

Unit-shared governance communication

New technology or practice education

Education for practice deficiency

Attendance at professional staff meetings

Is research a growing part of the units' activities involving the staff in research activities?

Compliance with the council research plan

Unit research priorities in conjunction with council plan

Format for disseminating research information

Accommodation of outside research

Application of research findings

Each unit must incorporate into its implementation plan at least the above considerations and their impact on the staff. Since these are assumed to be staff-driven processes in shared governance, it is important that they form the basis of the unit staff expression of their accountabilities in a shared governance framework. The following should be remembered: as much as possible shared governance activities should be done in the course of patient care in a shared governance format including the patient, where viable, in professional processes that affect care. As much as is possible, *shared governance activities at the unit level should not increase the workload or time commitment of the individual practitioner*. It is the expectation that the unit staff and management should attempt to incorporate much of the obligation for performance and participation in shared governance into their usual and normal workload and practice activities.

Initially, the manager may have to play a larger role in undertaking some of the first activities on the units related to shared governance. The tension here will relate to the contradiction between those activities the manager undertakes and the accountability for those actions that is supposed to emerge in the staff.

Like all change, often those who complete the change are not the ones who initiate it. A rule of implementation is to always use the rules in place at the time of initiation, not those hoped to replace the current structure. This will often mean that the more traditional approaches to getting things started might have to be used. When the contradiction becomes apparent to the staff and interferes with their ownership of the process, the manager will then know to pull back and simply facilitate the staff's development.

SPECIAL IMPLICATIONS FOR UNION ENVIRONMENTS

There is no reason why shared governance cannot be successful in union organized settings (see Chapter 9 in **Implementing Shared Governance**). There is a high level of compatibility between the values of shared governance and the elements of collective bargaining. Shared governance neither causes nor prevents the union organization of hospitals; it facilitates relationships within a work group and organizes the group based on the character of the relationship and the accountability for the work.

Much change is engendered in the workplace through the introduction of shared governance. Because it is a model that fundamentally alters the organization and roles in the workplace, it has an effect on all the players. Union members are not exempt from these changes. All relationships and structures are affected and will demand dialogue and negotiation to be successful. In many ways contract items and language will be affected by the design and function of shared governance. This should be no more threatening to the organization or the collective bargaining agents than any major social change occurring at this time. As organizations move toward the twenty-first century, all relationships will be affected as people retool their work structures and relationships to represent changing realities. A lack of flexibility in the face of these many social, economic, and technical changes diminishes the effectiveness and value of any group in getting ready for the future.

In union environments the following considerations must always form a part of the implementation process if the transformation to shared governance is to be successful:

> Union leadership must be involved in all phases of the development of shared governance from the outset.
>
> All issues identified in the contract are subject to discussion as they affect implementing shared governance.
>
> There are no hidden agendas in shared governance. Efforts to avoid generating them are encouraged.
>
> If the contract is implicated in a shared governance change, discussion between organization and union leadership must occur before the change is completed.

No change in economic or workplace issues as outlined in the contract should be affected without the agreement of the bargaining teams.

Shared governance as a structure should be supported within the language of the contract to indicate the strength of the commitment of the parties to the contract to shared governance.

Elements of the shared governance processes should not be included in contract language to provide as much flexibility in design and adjustments as necessary to assure effectiveness.

The Executive Council should have some relationship or representation to or from the union leadership to facilitate communication, relationship, and problem solving.

Shared governance changes the organization radically. If both parties to the collective bargaining process are either not aware of this factor or are unwilling to enter into this collective reorganization, it should not be attempted until they are in agreement with regard to initiating shared governance. Too much is at stake for the staff and management to enter into this degree of organizational restructuring without the support of all the players. Since unit level life of the worker is significantly altered by shared governance and empowerment changes many of the traditional characterizations of the roles of managers and staff, many of the "old" work delineators and values are not viable. Traditional master-servant and labor-management orientations are simply not adequate to the environment that shared governance engenders. Shared governance will create a new kind of relationship in the organization and will cause both union and management to rethink and restructure their interactions, roles, and relationships. All parties to the collective bargaining process should be prepared to understand this reality before implementing shared governance in their organizations (see also Chapter 9 in **Implementing Shared Governance**).

Implementing Change

In making any significant change, it can be expected that there will be challenges to all involved. The process of implementation of shared governance will take 3 to 5 years to complete. People should be prepared to spend at least this amount of time in the implementation process. All of the change factors that influence success will have an impact on the transitions associated with shared governance (see Chapter 6 in **Implementing Shared Governance**).

Perhaps the greatest challenge to implementation will be resistance to changing current activities and frames of reference. It will take creating "noise" in the system to bring the trauma of change to the fore. All life transitions, including those in the workplace, involve significant emotional response. Changing people's lives, even when needed, causes them to move from certainty (even when the certainty is itself dysfunctional) to ambivalent, equivocal, and nontrusting behaviors. This should be expected.

ENDINGS

Whenever there is change, some loss occurs. Staff and managers must deal with these losses. Generally three steps create a sense of endings in the staff and leadership. They are disengagement, disidentification, and disenchantment. To begin the process of change, a formal process must be entered into. People will go through the processes associated with the change in a systematic way, consistent with their needs and perception of its impact on them. The leader must be able to identify the stage and the behaviors that exemplify it.

Disengagement

There must be a significant shift that promises major adjustments in expectation and performance. Both the symbolic and the real must converge to create an emerging new reality so different that the old is no longer adequate in the emerging reality.

Understanding the need for a period of disengagement and incorporating it into the change process are essential for change to be successful. Issues related to the move to a new reality must be adequately addressed:

How is the new so different from the old?

N   O   T   E   S

What will be missed in the hierarchy that staff liked?

How will the changes alter our relationships?

What is different in the workplace in shared governance that is significant?
   1.

   2.

   3.

   4.

   5.

How does the change affect me personally?
   1.

   2.

   3.

What personal adjustments in my professional and personal life will occur as a result of shared governance?

    1.

    2.

    3.

Is our unit staff ready to pull together and build shared governance on the unit?

What gets in the way of our staff "getting started" with shared governance?

    1.

    2.

    3.

    4.

    5.

What supports the unit's move to shared governance?

    1.

N   O   T   E   S

2.

3.

4.

5.

What do I most hate/like about change?
    1.

    2.

What things will be the hardest for me to give up as we move to shared governance?
    1.

    2.

    3.

The staff and management will need to consciously disengage from old values. The above questions help identify the values and issues of a personal nature that each member of the staff confronts in making a change of this magnitude. Recognizing that creating new organizational models begins the writing of the script for the future. With no precedents for this enterprise, all the securities and assurances of the past slip away and the organization moves into ambiguity and even discord as it attempts to write its new script. With all the players involved, including the staff, it can become a noisy process. The leader will need to keep a close eye on the dynamics and the changes, always staying focused and moving the staff in a direction that can best meet the goals of a shared governance system.

Disidentification

As mentioned previously, a major shift in both structuring and operating the organization begins with the initiation of shared governance. The old behavioral "tapes" are played because they best represent what we know and apply in ways that once worked; but they are no longer adequate for the task of reformatting the organization. This is best identified as a paradigm shift. What occurs often reflects a way of thinking that challenges the old ways. Leadership and staff actually have to consciously deny the value of the tradition they are moving out of and apply a new set of values and principles as tests for their thinking and acting. They must disidentify with the traditional thinking and ways and begin to identify with the new.

Questions that address this change are often challenging and very specific:

What are the fundamental principles of shared governance?

   1.

   2.

   3.

   4.

   5.

   6.

   7.

<u>N   O   T   E   S</u>

8.

9.

10.

What do I have to believe in a shared governance workplace that was not necessary in the traditional framework?

What will this new model do for the profession; for each other; for me?

What "old ways" especially appeal to me or to which I am particularly attached?

What three elements of conflict between the old and the new ways are going to affect me the most?

1.

2.

3.

What old behaviors will I have to work hardest to consciously change to be effective in the shared governance framework?

The most important work in the process of disidentifying is to begin to identify with the new. The leader will have to become especially sensitive to the issues that get in the way of identifying with the new model. He or she will have to help staff identify beliefs and behaviors that prevent them from changing and teach them to adapt to behaviors that exemplify accountability and shared decision making.

Disenchantment

This important phase is the final step in initiating personal transition. As one finds that the old is no longer effective for the role and for personal success, movement away from what was once valued becomes easier. Disenchantment allows for the final separation from what was once valued and allows the new values and processes to become a part of one's expectation and life. Often it is expressed in the organization by those who cannot remember or understand what the old way was or how it operated. New behaviors that exemplify the values of the shared governance system begin to emerge and staff rejects those of the past.

It is important that the staff get through this phase. Failure to pass through disenchantment can result in bitterness and rejection. There are always staff members who are extremely reticent to undertake any major change. To be successful and to obtain compliance, their issues will have to be addressed and their reality orientation will need adjustment. If this is not dealt with, there can be much obstreperous behavior and mixed efforts to sabotage the changes and even the whole concept of shared governance.

The leader should assess the status of the staff as they move through the separation from their more traditional behaviors. Of course, each member of the staff will move at a different rate. For this reason, the change agent would have an awareness of each person's adaptation and monitor it individually. Usually there are definitive behavioral changes that are sought out and are characteristic of the specific change. They can become the indicators for the change agent and the means of assessing where individuals are in making their own transition.

RESISTANCE TO CHANGE

Resistance to change is a natural and normative process in humans. However, change is the only constant in the universe. Learning to anticipate and then undertake the appropriate action reflective of the change is the challenge of life.

Because of this dichotomy, it is essential that a culture of acceptance of change, even an anticipation of it, is necessary in the organization. Introducing shared governance is such an important change with a great deal of structural revision occurring that a commitment to what the change implies is essential to its long-term success.

Some reasons for resistance to organizational change are these:

Old routines; old habits
Laziness
Comfort
Fear
Costs of change
Threat to existing relationships
Inadequate leadership
Poor change climate
Traditional successes

Awareness of the specific resistance factors the leader will confront will assist in strategy development for making the necessary changes. Each organization will have its own complex factors influencing its ability to implement the shared governance process. The leader should be aware of the institution's unique culture and identify strategies for addressing them.

CHANGE AGENTS

The change agent role is essential to the transition to shared governance. In almost any organization there is a person that operates as the agent of change. This person is often the catalyst and moderator of the change. In a shared governance effort, this person need not be the manager, although it usually starts out with the manager as facilitator of change.

Whoever plays the role, he or she will use a number of approaches to make the change and should be aware of the context of these models so that they might be consciously applied:

Consciousness raiser: This role focuses on the issues that appear to be a contest in the organization. This person asks the why questions and raises the inadequacies of the status quo. He or she articulates what everyone recognizes but did not give form. These people do not accept the status quo and tend to make everyone uncomfortable with great equality. This person will use the following technique to initiate change:
  Questions
  Identifies problems
  Points out issues
  Identifies dissatisfiers
  Identifies possible changes
  Challenges authority
  Is politically assertive

Implementor: This person is less concerned with the issues than the processes involved in making changes. He or she is interested in constructing processes that can give form to undertaking change and moving along the continuum of change. He or she is best characterized by the following:
  Defines the need for change
  Identifies possible ways of responding
  Looks at ways of changing
  Generates ideas
  Tries to stimulate interest

Outcome seeker: this person seeks the results of the effort for change. She has usually accepted the fact that change is going to occur and now looks more toward what will be produced as a result of the change and seeks to identify what that will look like. She usually exhibits the following characteristics:
  Goal orientation
  Solution finder
  Bottom line orientation
  Wants behavior change
  Anxious to get there
  Impatient
  Task based

Linkage creator: This leader is committed to the success of the transition and recognizes that the change makers cannot arrive at their change alone. The relationship they establish and the others they touch in the process are important to its success. They also seek to link resources to the project to ensure that it has what it needs to succeed. Some of the attributes of this person are these:
  Establishes good relationships
  Forms coalitions

Is politically aware

Is fiscally proficient

Finds resources

Balancer: This leader keeps all in a sense of equilibrium. She stabilizes the environment and moderates against the noise of change. She brings order and meaning to the change. This leader can take the efforts to date and formalize them and assure that they operate as planned. The old is over and the change agent can simply entrench the new and deal with the issues of normalizing the work environment. Some of the characteristics of this person are:

Defines the boundaries

Creates relationships

Builds solidarity

Establishes new values

Normalizes the environment

Conceives linkages

It should be clear to the leader that these change agents all have different skills and roles to play in undertaking change. They are all necessary to the change process and will be valuable in implementing shared governance but each at different times and in different ways.

THE CHANGE PROCESS

The implementor and innovator should always have a model for implementing change. This is no less true for shared governance implementation. Change models give form to the change process and a plan and timetable for assessing progress and evaluating change. A formal process allows the participants to note progress and to see change, thus keeping the change process on course and organized.

Every change agent should undertake to plan the steps in the process and complete a time line for implementation. They should be able to break down the major components of implementation and define the action steps necessary to stay on course and achieve the anticipated outcomes. As mentioned earlier in this workbook, it will take anywhere from 3 to 5 years to implement shared governance depending on the degree of commitment and the structures in place. The time line should reflect that reality.

The following questions provide an initial framework for beginning to put some form to a plan:

Generally, how well understood is the concept of shared governance?

Has the planning group been formed?

What is the ultimate outcome of shared governance?

What initial model is selected?

What has already happened to provide support for shared governance?

How large is your organization?

What resources are available to the implementation team?

What change model has been selected to evaluate progress?

What level of interest exists and where has it been generated initially?

Where are the managers in their understanding and commitment?

What educational programming and resources will be required?

While this is not an exhaustive list of issues, it does help the planner put some form to his or her thinking and begin to pull some of the pieces together.

It should be remembered that few plans end up in precisely the same way in which they were conceived. Planning provides a framework for action. The vagaries of change and the many influences on process have a striking impact on how the finished product will appear. There are many influences along the way that will determine the eventual design and outcome of the shared governance transition. The leader should not be locked into rigid parameters in planning. Instead, the plan should simply provide the guidelines that moderate and monitor progress along a continuum.

Whatever approach is taken, the leadership must identify the model for change that they will use in the unfolding of the shared governance process. All of the group processes that are directed to the implementation of shared governance should be incorporated into the change model selected.

PRELIMINARY RESEARCH

It is recommended that some preliminary baseline be established before shared governance implementation is undertaken. Also, the process should be examined along the way for progress and the relationship of the process to its outcomes. Issues related to staff satisfaction, organizational design, motivation, cost, change in expectation, impact on service and other service providers, and consistency with the mission of the setting are all appropriate arenas for establishing a base line. Of course, the organization should also have individualized goals it would like to see addressed by shared governance processes. There are a number of resources available to the individual institution already constructed and identified in the literature, (see Appendix A). Each institution, however, should be encouraged to undertake the design of instruments of their own to determine data that are specific to its own needs or directed to a specific purpose.

Since implementation of shared governance is a process that will take some time, it is important to establish several times in which the process and its outcomes will be studied over the period of implementation. Usually implementing shared governance takes a full 5 years to complete. However, various outcomes are usually achieved along the way and behavioral change can be noted. Undertaking studies that relate to the nature and the degree of change helps the leadership assess where they are and the aspect of change or transition needing more attention and/or readiness for the next phase of development. The usual period of time for study is about once a year during the phases of implementation. The phases as identified in this work book and the text **Implementing Shared Governance** could be identified as follows:

Conception
Initiation
Design
Formation
Structuring
Formalization
Perpetuation

These seven phases are generally complete in the 5 years of transition. Those that are interested in doing detailed research about any or all of the phases could look at structuring research projects at increments that would best demarcate these phases. The best approach, however, is to establish a calendar time frame for structuring studies, ensuring a clearer, more definitive time context for measurement. The important point is that the studies of process and impact should occur as early as possible in implementation.

EMPOWERMENT PROCESS

Just because shared governance brings a professional milieu to life and empowers both the professional and the profession, it does not guarantee that the staff are going to race to shared governance in great numbers at the outset (refer to Chapter 3 in **Implementing Shared Governance**). The process of empowerment changes what has become the expectation in the workplace built over 90 years of formation. In addition, the prevailing social norms and expectations often moderate against many of the notions and ideals that comprise the shared governance concept. It should be anticipated that there will be many questions and concerns from all levels of the organization regarding the value and efficacy of shared governance. The long history of employer-employee thinking and organizational formation will not easily give way to the partnership processes and partnering in the workplace. Old realities die hard, especially when one group receives the advantage, often at the disadvantage of another. Both groups, however, learn their roles well and find it difficult to change them even when they might want to change what they imply.

Implementing shared governance implies, however, that the work of changing this reality will begin and the parties will undertake the work of changing their work and their relationship with each other (see Chapter 6 in **Implementing Shared Governance**). This, too, will have to be a process that unfolds new descriptors of relationship and accountability as those both change throughout the implementation process. The process of empowerment demands commitment from all parties and will result in significant changes for all who are involved and invested in it.

STRUCTURAL CHANGES

In order to successfully implement shared governance, the organization will have to expect that the following structures will undergo major change in the transforming activities that lead to mutuality and empowerment.

Multidisciplinary work flow patterns
Open-ended communication structures
Continuous assessment of work patterns
Universal access to resources
Investment at all levels of the workplace
Growing dependence on interdependence
Change in role definitions
Movement away from status determinations
Accountability basis, not hierarchy

ORGANIZATIONAL CHANGES

An empowered work place has more organizational structuring, which affords an unlimited approach to relationships and rewards. Newer consciousness regarding how relationships are structured and how work is rewarded will have to be considered. Some challenges are the following:

All salaried work roles
Alternative reward systems
Gainsharing strategies
Clarity of role accountability
Partnership mentality
Mentoring roles
Variable loci of leadership roles
Work achievement-reward systems
Work redesign (worker driven)
New orientation/socialization processes

Clearly these characteristics will not emerge automatically or without some deeply considered deliberation and planning. However, these do change the character of work and relationships and transform the workplace and the relationships that produce work outcomes. Openness to such changes and adaptations by owners, managers, and staff is vital to successful workplace transformation.

CULTURAL CHANGES

A formalized approach to making a significant change will have to be determined. In addition to the specific service-based management changes identified for the Management Council earlier in this workbook, there needs to be a structured approach to teaching the development of a new cultural awareness in the workplace. The following items identify some of those elements that will reflect this change:

Altered reward systems
Continuous management development
Continuous leadership development (manager and staff)
Career enhancement programs
Staff hiring and termination processes
Staff role ownership (including position descriptions)
Creative benefits programs
Unit of service programs instead of divisional ones

It is easy to see that the empowerment process depends on a new way of thinking, indeed a new paradigm for the leaders and manager of the workplace. No small effort is involved in making this change. It calls for a complete openness to retooling the workplace with new thinking, new roles, and different approaches to rewards and relationships.

INDIVIDUAL CHANGES

Structures and efforts that lead to empowered behaviors in the professional worker must be applied to successfully achieve changed behaviors. These programs should begin at the unit or service level and be a part of the education and developmental work of the leadership of each unit. As identified in previous sections of this workbook, a unit-based approach to changing employee behaviors will have to be concerted and planned. The staff will not know to want the change and may reject it at the outset. Incorporated into their work and the expectations of role and relationship should be changed structure and thus changed behavior as reinforced by the changed structure. Developmental activities should be directed in a formalized way to produce active and responsive behaviors.

Individual responsibility also means that changes will occur in the staff. At some time staff will have to make the requisite changes that all professionals will have to exhibit in a partnership organization and a professional enterprise. Again, how those changes are made will depend specifically on the culture and the particular characteristics of the organization. While this workbook is helpful in identifying the specific changes and can outline the requisite characteristics and stages of change, it would take an encyclopedic effort to enumerate all of the necessary change strategies for each culture and unit here. There are many fine resources available to the change agent, including those listed in Appendix A, which can be an excellent resource for the change agent.

Some of the behaviors that exemplify the staff transition follow:

Openness to new realities
Willingness to change
Sound practice standards
Clear sense of ethics
Openness to dialogue issues
Fundamental honesty
Emerging curiosity
Willingness to seek concensus
Ability to express concerns
Structured risk taking (safer)
Commitment to competency
Willingness to abide by concensus
Varying degree of involvement
Growing toward self-esteem
Varying levels of creativity

The staff member will experience the greatest level of personal change. Impact on the individual role will be the greatest result of the changes in the workplace. Therefore a growing awareness of the emerging changes and a transformation of his or her motivation and commitment will evidence the success of the change strategies and their impact on his or her life.

Questions for every staff member relate to their willingness to experience the transformation in their own personal lives and practice:

How open am I to major changes when they affect me? (I have to change.)

List three kinds of personal change I dislike the most
     1.

     2.

     3.

What behaviors arise in me when I have to undertake change I do not like?

What is my greatest source of satisfaction in my work?

How would I characterize my obligation to my peers in the work place?

What do I think is their obligation to me?

Do I think changes in the way I work and my relationships at work are inevitable?

How do I perceive my leadership role?

How do I manifest my leadership role at work?

What does personal transformation mean to me?

How do I perceive my manager's role in undertaking major change at work?

What does it mean to me to act in an empowered way?

What are my three greatest strengths as a person?
    1.

    2.

    3.

N   O   T   E   S

My three major areas of personal growth?

    1.

    2.

    3.

What other roles in my life affect my ability and time to participate more fully in work-related activities?

What are my personal career goals?

    Education

    Timetable

    Work

    Timetable

Career advancement

Timetable

Role changes

Timetable

How do my personal goals coincide with the changing realities affecting my profession? My work? My personal life?

All change will demand a personal commitment sometime in the process by all those affected by the change. Getting the staff involved in their part of the process as they are able and at a time of preparedness will be vital to the success of any change. As indicated above, not all staff will be ready for change at the same time. Raising consciousness, as attempted by the above questions, can facilitate the timing and the processing of change. When tied to the questions related to implementing shared governance earlier in this workbook, they can provide a catalyst for initiating change.

Implementing Bylaws

Bylaws are usually the last of the formal shared governance activities directly related to implementing shared governance. Many organizations begin with formatting the bylaws and let them provide the direction and guidelines for the implementation of shared governance. The problem with this approach is that bylaws are generally descriptive tools, describing what is already in place in the organization. When they are used as developmental tools, they are continually revised and take up valuable time that should really be spent in developmental work. Sometimes developing bylaws can even serve as a diversionary tactic during tough times in implementation when "hot issues" need to be addressed directly and it is not safe to do so for whatever reason. Focusing on bylaws, however, never resolved an issue that needed dialogue and group effort to confront directly.

It is usually wiser to use a developmental plan for the process of implementation instead of bylaws. To do so more directly addresses the process and helps keep the concept and content of bylaws free of the controversies associated with development. Bylaws are best used when they describe what is already in place and provide a framework for understanding and managing the shared governance process.

Generally the ExC constructs and manages the bylaws (see Chapter 8 in **Implementing Shared Governance**). Since they are responsible for maintaining the integrity of the system and ensuring that the system operates as it should, they are most often the formulators and controllers of the bylaws. Once the bylaws are formulated, the ExC must approve any staff request for a bylaws change before it can go to the staff annual meeting for general vote of approval. This provides checks and balances to assure the bylaws are not arbitrarily changed or altered by individual members or groups of members of the staff without a rational review of how they affect the integrity of the professional organization and how they affect the way it does its work.

Bylaws are essential because they more adequately and professionally define the relationships and operational characteristics of a professional group in a way different from a vocational or technical work group in the organization. Bylaws indicate that the discipline recognizes the inherent ownership of its work and the aggregate obligation the profession has to serve the public in its unique manner consistent with the law and social madate that is reflected in their accountability. The bylaws should express this reality and give evidence of it in the way in which they are constructed. Both the public and the institution have a right to expect that the best interests of the service receiver are addressed within the resource constraints of the service setting.

Bylaws should also be thorough in their presentation of how the professional organization operates. As more of the professional disciplines are drawn into shared governance approaches, there will be less need for divisional bylaws that are exclusive in their coverage and a greater need for inclusive bylaws that address the corporate professional relations in the organization with specified rules and regulations for each of the disciplines. This concern, however, is some distance away. Usually, few disciplines begin the shared governance process and are therefore formative in their efforts. Usually it is the nursing service that most often begins the process of implementation with other professional services beginning at a later date. It will be some years in most institutions before the need for an aggregate approach to professional bylaws emerge in more than a very few settings.

ELEMENTS OF THE BYLAWS

Bylaws' articles are fairly generic and consistent in all professional organizations or bodies. Shared governance bylaws are very similar in this regard. The articles compose the main delineators and provide the format for the sections and subsections of the bylaws format.

Major articles usually fall into the following categories (see sample bylaws in Appendix F):

Article 1
Preamble
  Section 1—Purpose of the bylaws
  Section 2—Definition of practice
  Section 3—Conceptual basis for practice
  Section 4—Philosophy of the discipline
  Section 4—Purpose of the discipline
  Section 5—Critical objectives of the service

Article 2
  Role of the Professional
    Section 1—Role of the discipline
    Section 2—Role of the member
    Section 3—Professional expectations

Article 3
  Major Clinical Services
    Section 1—Major clinical services
    Section 2—Organization of the services
    Section 3—Disciplines covered by these bylaws

Article 4
  Professional Staff Membership
    Section 1—Definition of membership
    Section 2—Definition of the professional staff
    Section 3—Conditions of and duration of appointment to the professional staff
    Section 4—Eligibility for appointment to the professional staff
    Section 5—Other categories of appointment
    Section 6—Provisional appointment process
    Section 7—Credentials review process
    Section 8—Rejection of appointment of candidate by the professional staff
    Section 9—Appeals process related to failure to be appointed to professional staff

Article 5
  Governance Structure of the Professional Staff
    Section 1—Definition of the governance bodies, (councils)
    Section 2—Membership on governance body

Section 3—Role of each body
Section 4—Responsibility of governance body members
Section 5—Responsibility of the governance body chair
Section 6—Role and function of the Executive Body
Section 7—Meeting time and format of governance bodies
Section 8—Section of governance body members
Section 9—Service and tenure of governance body members

Article 6

Discipline, Appeals, Advancement, Performance Review, and Removal from the Professional Staff
Section 1—Disciplinary action process
Section 2—Professional appeals process
Section 3—Review process for advancement
Section 4—Performance review processes
Section 5—Procedure for removal from the professional staff

Article 7

Coordination of the Professional Staff and Management of the Clinical Service
Section 1—Role of management in the professional organization
Section 2—Role of the service executive in the professional organization
Section 3—Coordination of the executive and governance functions in the professional organization
Section 4—Role, time, and function of the quarterly professional staff meetings
Section 5—Role, time, and function of the annual professional staff meeting

Article 8

Bylaw Revision
Section 1—Articles
Section 2—Executive body control
Section 3—Revision
Section 4—Amendments
Section 5—Annual review

Article 9

Rules and Regulations
Section 1—Professional rules
Section 2—Service rules and regulations
Section 3—Governance body approval of rules and regulations

Article 10

Adoption of the Bylaws

The above items of the bylaws will contain the specific information related to the operation of the professional staff and the organization. All of the elements of the coordination of a professional body in an institution and a work group are included in the articles and sections of the bylaws. There are no standard inclusions in the sections of the bylaws. Each organization must represent its unique approach and model in the descriptors incorporated in the bylaws.

The bylaws should be as detailed and complete as possible. They should briefly but thoroughly cover the key operational and governance issues affecting the smooth and efficient operation of the professional organization. They are a challenge to construct. It is sometimes difficult to adequately and concisely describe the meaning and nuances of the professional staff and organization. Relationships and accountability, however, depend on the accuracy and thoroughness of the contents of the bylaws. Remember also that every member of the staff and management of the organization will use the bylaws as the operational and relational guide for both operations and problem solving. Decision-making structures and strategies will reflect the accountabilities and functions that are articulated within the bylaws.

Bylaws construction takes 6 months to a year of focused work by the executive council or designated body. It is recommended that they be reviewed by an attorney for content, language, and a review of their implications within the existing body of employer-employee law (labor relations). It must be remembered, however, that you are writing a new script for organizing professional work and relationships in the work place: current law covering the work place may not be adequate to the new descriptors and relationships that emerge in creating a shared governance organizational system.

The bylaws should, when completed and approved by the staff and management of the professional organization, have the approval of the administration and board of the institution. As the staff enter into a new kind of relationship with the workplace and articulate it in the organizational structure and the bylaws, the corporate leadership has a right to participate in a review and approval of it within the context of their governance obligation for the system. With their approval, the bylaws then become an important part of the structure of the organization and now have the governance support of the board and administration of the organization. This commitment then represents the partnership between the institution and the professions that do the work of health care. It is this partnership that exemplifies the central value of the shared governance approach.

CHANGED CULTURE

Change of the kind outlined in this workbook will result in a significantly altered workplace and culture of work. The workplace will become much more dynamic and fluid, responding more easily to changing demands and changing structures. There results a much broader orientation to accountability and corporate responsibility, indeed, a stronger commitment to it. There is a stronger merger between the individual and the community of work with less differentiation than the present "us-them" framework. Increase in horizontal communication and decision making results in a higher level of ownership by all and increasing level of mutuality with regard to both work and relationships.

The demarcation between worker and manager, while still very clear, is less so by status than by role and accountability. The trust-based interaction of each with the other receives renewed emphasis and creates an understanding of the contributions of the other.

As indicated in this workbook and the text, **Implementing Shared Governance,** the processes associated with implementation of the shared governance concept are more vehicle than outcome. The shared governance process indicates a philosophy, an approach to work and relationships that builds a community committed to mutual processes and outcomes. These processes in shared governance reflect the value and trust necessary to real success instead of unilateral outcomes that may reflect economic viability for some at the expense of true social growth and enhancement in the quality of life of all the participants. In that effort, even the characteristics of shared governance outlined in this workbook and the accompanying text are subject to transformation and change. This is as it should be. The processes of our collective growth must reflect that growth in their own elements. In this way they facilitate our development instead of encouraging it at the outset only to impede it later on. The principles, however, remain the same. It is in emphasizing the principles of community, mutuality, and empowerment that shared governance takes its form. It is to that end this workbook is directed.

Bibliography

This bibliography contains a large body of information that may be helpful in the formation of shared governance concepts and in the implementation of shared governance models. Some of the literature is foundational, going back to the body of knowledge on which the concept is based. This foundational literature is provided for those who wish to substantiate the body of knowledge supporting the move to shared governance as being both legitimate and timely.

Also listed are those authors who are beginning to envision newer models for doing work and organizing the American workplace to renew its vitality and viability on the global stage. Much of the material in this arena is visionary and needs to be validated by extensive research activities. Some is currently in the process of research exploration. Since we are in a transforming world, the state of the available information supporting partnerships in the workplace is emerging at a quantum rate. The reader and implementor of shared governance should be sensitive to the relevant literature and add resources to this bibliography as they become available.

The leaders in developing shared governance approaches should expand their frames of reference regarding the available literature in shared governance. Much new work is emerging in almost all fields of human science. While the professional literature is valuable to the clinical professional, reading in organizations, human resources, psychology of work, and work redesign will add to the individual's understanding of changes in the workplace and in shared governance.

Abell P: Hierarchy and democratic authority. In Burns TR et al: Work and power, Beverly Hills, Calif, 1979, Sage Publications Inc.

Adams J: Tranforming work, Alexandria, Va, 1984, Miles River Press.

Aiken LH and Mullinix CF: Special report: The nursing shortage—myth or reality? N Engl J Med 317(10):641-645, 1986.

Alward, R: Nursing administration in crisis, Nurs Forum 19(3):243-253, 1980.

American Academy of Nursing: Magnet hospitals' attraction and retention of professional nurses, Kansas City, Mo, 1983, American Nurses Association.

American Hospital Association: Profile of the nursing service administrator revisited, Unpublished report, Chicago, 1980, The Association.

American Hospital Association: Role, function, and qualifications of the nursing service administrator in a health care institution, Chicago, 1979, The Association.

American Nurses Association: Nursing: a social policy statement, Kansas City, Mo, 1980, The Association.

American Nurses Association: Standards for nursing services, Kansas City, Mo, 1974, The Association.

American Society for Nursing Service Administrators: Preparation of nurse managers: informational bulletin, Chicago, 1979, The Society.

Archer SE and Goehner PA: Nurses: a political force, North Scituate, Mass, 1981, Wadsworth Health Sciences Division.

Argyris C: Interpersonal competence and organizational effectiveness, Homewood, Ill, 1962, Irwin Dorsey Press.

Argyris C: Teaching smart people how to learn, Harvard Bus Rev 69(3):99-109, 1991.

Ashley J: About power in nursing, Nurs Outlook 21(10):641, 1973.

Athos A and Coffey R: Behavior in organizations: a multidimensional view, Englewood Cliffs, NJ, 1968, Prentice-Hall.

Baird JE Jr: Changes in nurse attitudes: management strategies for today's environment, J Nurs Adm 17(9):109-120, 1987.

Bajnok IJ and Gitterman G: Nurses as colleagues and mentors, Can Nurse 84:16-17, 1988.

Baker C: Moving toward interdependence strategies for collaboration, Nurse Educator pp 27-31, September-October 1981.

Barhyte DY, Counte M, and Christman L: The effects of decentralization on nurses' job attendance behaviors, Nurs Adm Q 11(4):37-46, 1987.

Beecroft P: A contractual model for the department of nursing, J Nurs Adm 18(9):20-24, 1988.

Belenky MF et al: Women's ways of knowing: the development of self, voice, and mind, New York, 1986, Basic Books.

Benner P: From novice to expert, Menlo Park, Calif, 1984, Addison-Wesley Publishing Co.

Bennis W: Beyond bureaucracy: essays on the development and evolution of human organizations, New York, 1973, McGraw-Hill Book Co.

Bennis W: On becoming a leader, New York, 1989, Addison-Wesley Publishing Co.

Bennis W and Benne K: The planning of change, New York, 1976, Holt, Rinehart & Winston.

Bennis W and Nanus B: Leaders: the strategies for taking charge, New York, 1985, Harper & Row.

Benveniste G: Professionalizing the organization, San Francisco, 1987, Jossey-Bass.

Berne E: Games people play, New York, 1964, Grove Press.

Beyers M: Leadership in nursing, Wakefield, Mass, 1979, Nursing Resources.

Binger J and Huntsman A: Coaching: a technique to increase employee performance, AORN J 47:229-233, 1988.

Blair E: Needed, nursing administration leaders, Nurs Outlook 21(10):641, 1973.

Blake R, editor: Perception: an approach to personality, New York, 1951, Roandel Press.

Blake R and Mouton J: The managerial grid, Houston, 1964, Gulf Publishing.

Blazeck A et al: Unification: nursing education and nursing practice, Nurs Health Care, pp 18-24, January 1982.

Booth RZ: Power: a negative or positive force in relationships? Nurs Adm Q 7(4):10-20, 1983.

Boyle RJ: Wrestling with jellyfish, Harvard Bus Rev 61(1):74-83, 1984.

Bracken R and Christman L: An incentive program designed to reward clinical competence, J Nurs Adm 10:8-18, 1978.

Braun K et al: Verbal abuse of nurses and non nurses, Nurs Management 22(3):72-76, 1991.

Brenner P and Wrubel J: The primary of caring: stress and coping in health and illness, Menlo Park, Calif, 1989, Addison-Wesley Publishing Co.

Brittan A and Maynard M: Sexism, racism and oppression, London, 1984, Basil Blackwell.

Burke GC III: Renewal and change for health care executives, Hosp Health Serv Adm 36(1):13-23, 1991.

Bylaws, St. Mary's Hospital and Health Center, 1987, Tucson, Ariz.

Callahan CB and Wall LL: Participative management: a contingency approach, J Nurs Adm 17:9-15, 1987.

Cantor RM: When giants learn to dance, New York, 1989, Simon & Schuster.

Capers CF: Using nursing models to guide nursing practice: key questions, J Nurs Adm 16(11):40-43, 1986.

Capers CF et al: The Neuman systems model in practice: planning phase, J Nurs Adm 15(5):29-39, 1985.

Caramanica L and Thibodeau J: Staff involvement in developing a nursing philosophy and selection of a model for practice, Nurs Management 18(10):71, 1987.

Cartwright D and Zander A, editors: Group dynamics: research and theory, Evanston, Ill, 1960, Row Peterson & Co.

Champoux JE: A three sample test of some extensions of the job characteristics model of work motivation, Acad Management J 23(3):466-478, 1980.

Chaska N: The nursing profession: turning points, St Louis, 1990, The CV Mosby Co.

Christman L: Accountability and autonomy are more than rhetoric, Nurse Educator 3:3-6, 1978.

Cialdini RB: Influence: how and why people agree to things, New York, 1984, William Morrow & Co, Inc.

Ciancutti A et al: Creating harmony between supervisor and nurse, Supervisor Nurse 7(3):33-37, 1976.

Cleland VS: Nurses' economics and the control of nursing practice. In Aiden L, editor: Nursing in the 1980's, Philadelphia, 1982, JB Lippincott Co.

Cleland VS: Shared goverance in a professional model of collective bargaining, J Nurs Adm 8:39-42, 1978.

Clifford J: Managerial control versus professional autonomy: a paradox, J Nurs Adm 11:19-21, 1981.

Colton M: Nursing leadership vacuum, Supervisor Nurse, pp 29-37, October 1976.

Cowart ME: Teaching the legislative process, Nurs Outlook 25:777-780, 1977.

Cox H: Verbal abuse in nursing: report of a study, Nurs Management 18(11):47-50, 1987.

Cox H: Verbal abuse nationwide. Part II. Impact and modifications, Nurs Management 22(3):66-69, 1991.

Curtin KL: Professional collegiality, Supervisor Nurse 11:7, 1980.

Curtin LL: Autonomy, accountability and nursing practice, Topics Clin Nurs 5, 1982.

Dayani E: Professional and economic self-governance in nursing, Nurs Economics 1:20-23, 1983.

Deal TA and Kennedy AA: Corporate cultures: the rites and rituals of corporate life, Reading, Mass, 1982, Addison-Wesley Publishing Co.

delBueno D: Rational irrationality: an organizational alternative, J Nurs Adm 21(1):7-10, 1991.

Deloughery G and Gebbie K: Political dynamics: impact on nurses and nursing, St Louis, 1975, The CV Mosby Co.

Deming WE: Out of the crisis, Cambridge, 1986, Massachusetts Institute of Technology.

Dennis KE: Nursing's power in the organization, what research has shown nursing, Adm Q 8(2):47-56, 1983.

Deremo D: Integrating professional values: quality practice, productivity, and reimbursement for nursing, Nurs Adm Q 1:9-23, 1989.

Diers D: When college grads choose nursing, Am J Nurs 87(12):1631-1637, 1987.

Douglass LM and Bevis EO: Nursing management and leadership in action, St Louis, 1983, The CV Mosby Co.

Drucker P: Management, New York, 1974, Harper & Row.

Drucker P: Management: tasks, responsibility and practice, New York, 1973, Harper & Row.

Duffy M and Gold N: Education for nursing administration: What investment yields highest returns, Nurs Adm Q 5(1):31-32, 1980.

Durbin E and Zuckerman S: Legislation affects nursing practice, Nurs Adm Q 1:39-50, 1978.

Ecton DR and Fralic MF: Leadership in a changing environment, J Nurs Adm 17(12):6-9, 1987.

Egeland JW and Brown JS: Sex role stereotyping and role strain of male registered nurses, Res Health 11:257-267, 1988.

Elliott E: A discourse of nursing; A case of silencing, Nurs Healthcare 10(10):539-543, 1990.

Erickson E: The hospital nursing service administrator, doctoral dissertation, New York, 1972, Columbia University.

Erickson E: The nursing service director 1880-1980, J Nurs Adm, April 1980, pp 6-12.

Estok J: Socialization theory and entry into the practice of nursing, Image 9(1):13, 1977.

Ethridge P: As I see it: nursing centers make nursing care accessible, Am Nurs, pp 5-6, January 1987.

Ethridge P: Nurse accountability program improves satisfaction, turnover, Health Progress, pp 44-49, May 1987.

Fagin CM: Nurses for the future, Am J Nurs 87(12):1594-1595, 1987.

Ferguson M: The aquarian conspiracy, Los Angeles, 1980, Tarcher.

Fiedler F: Improving leadership effectiveness, New York, 1976, McGraw-Hill Book Co.

Fiedler F, Hutchins EB, and Dodge J: Psychological monographs, No. 473, Champaign, 1973, University of Illinois.

Flarey, DL: Redesigning management roles, J Nurs Adm 21(2):39-46, 1991.

Foster R: Innovation, New York, 1986, Summit.

Ganong W and Ganong J: Reducing organizational conflict through working committees, J Nurs Adm, Jan/Feb 1972.

Gardner JW: Excellence, New York, 1984, WW Norton.

Geus AP: Planning as learning, Harvard Bus Rev 66(2):70-74, 1988.

Gentleman C: Power at the unit level, Nurs Adm Q 7(2):27-31, 1982.

Ginzberg E: Nurses for the future: facing the facts and figures, Am J Nurs 87(12):1596-1600, 1987.

Goodrich N: A study of the competencies needed for nursing administration, doctoral dissertation, Washington, DC, 1981, George Washington University.

Gorman S and Clark N: Power and effective nursing practice, Nurs Outlook 34(3):129-134, 1986.

Grunwuld H: The second American century, Time, pp 70-75, October 8, 1990.

Haddad A: The nurses' role and responsibility in corporate level planning, Nurs Adm Q 5(2):1-3, 1981.

Hampton D: Behavioral concepts in management, Belmont, Calif, 1968, Dickinson Publishing Co.

Harding S: The science in feminism, Ithaca NY, 1986, Cornell University.

Herrick N: Joint management and employee participation, San Francisco, 1990, Jossey-Bass Inc.

Hersey P and Blanchard K: Management of organizational behavior: utilizing human resources, Englewood Cliffs, NJ, 1972, Prentice-Hall, Inc.

Hersey P, Blanchard K, and LaMonica E: A situational approach to supervision, Supervisor Nurse, pp 24-29, May 1976.

Herzburg F: Work and the nature of man, New York, 1966, World Publishing Co.

Hill B: The McAuley experience with changing compensation within the context of a professional nursing practice culture, Nurs Adm Q 14(1):78-82, 1989.

Hinshaw AS et al: Testing a theoretical model for job satisfaction and anticipated turnover of nursing staff (abstract), Nurs Res 34(6):384, 1985.

Hoerr J: What should unions do? Harvard Bus Rev 69(3):30-46, 1991.

Huckabay L: Point of view: nursing service and education. Is there a chasm? Nurs Adm Q 4(1):51-54, 1979.

Huey F and Harley S: What keeps nurses in nursing, Am J Nurs 88(2):181-188, 1988.

Johns Hopkins's nurses earn salaries and pursue autonomy in new professional practice units, Am J Nurs 87(5):713, 1987.

Johnson J: The education/service split. Who loses? Nurs Outlook 1:412-415, 1980.

Johnson L: A climate for survival. In Hanson RL, editor: Management systems for nursing service staffing, Rockville, Md, 1983, Aspen Publications.

Johnson L, Happel J and Edelman J: A model of participatory management with decentralized authority, Nurs Adm Q 8:30-36, 1983.

Johnston WB: Global work force 2000: The new world labor market, Harvard Bus Rev 69(3):115-127, 1991.

Jongewood D: Everybody wins: transactional analysis applied to organizations, Reading, Mass, 1973, Addison-Wesley Publishing Co.

Kaiser L: Visionary manager. In Wilson TC, editor: Emerging issues in health care 1988, Inglewood, Colo.

Kanter RM: The change masters: innovations and entrepreneurship, New York 1983, Simon & Schuster.

Kelman HC: Compliance, identification and internalization: three processes of attitude change, Conflict Resolution II, pp 51-60, 1958.

Kerfoot K: Managing professionals: the ultimate contradiction for nurse managers, Nurs Economics 6:321-322, 1988.

Kerfoot KM: Nursing management considerations, Nurs Economics 9(2):121-125, 1991.

Ketefian S: Professional and bureaucratic role conceptions and moral behavior among nurses, Nurs Res 34(4):248-253, 1985.

Kiesler C, Collins B, and Miller N: Attitude change: a critical analysis of theoretical approaches, New York, 1969, John Wiley & Sons.

Klein J: Why supervisors resist employee involvement, Harvard Bus Rev 61(1):87-95, 1984.

Kramer M: The magnet hospitals: excellence re-visited, J Nurs Adm 20(9):35-44, 1990.

Krejci JW and Malin S: A paradigm shift to the new age of nursing, Nurs Adm Q 13(4), 1989.

Lasay L and Maciariello J: Executive leadership in health care, San Francisco, 1991, Jossey-Bass Inc.

Law regulation—the practice of registered nursing, Olympia, 1974, State of Washington.

Lawrence JC: Confronting nurses' political apathy, Nurs Forum 15:363, 1976.

Leebov W: Healthcare managers in transition, San Francisco, 1990, Jossey-Bass Inc.

Lenninger M: Leadership crisis in nursing, J Nurs Adm, pp 28-34, March/April 1974.

Levenson A: The challenge of personal growth, Supervisor Nurse 8(11):66-67, 1977.

Levinson R: Knowledge of professional nursing legislation, Nurs Times 73:674-676, 1977.

Lewin K: Frontiers in group dynamics: concept, method and reality in social science: social equilibrium and social change, Hum Rel I (1):5-41, 1947.

Lewis FM and Batey MV: Clarifying autonomy and accountability in nursing service, Part 2, J Nurs Adm, pp 10-15, October 1982.

Likert R: The human organization, New York, 1967, McGraw-Hill Book Co.

Likert R: New patterns of management, New York, 1961, McGraw-Hill Book Co.

Lovell MC: Silent but perfect partners, medicine's use and abuse of women, Adv Nurs Sci 33(2):25-40, 1981.

Ludemann R and Brown C: Staff perceptions of shared governance, Nurs Adm Q 14(2):34-39, 1989.

Lun J: WICHEN, Panel of expert consultants report: implications for nursing leaders, J Nurs Adm, p 11, July 1979.

Lynaugh J: Nurses for the future: the yo-yo ride, Am J Nurs 87(12):1621-1630, 1987.

Lynch D and Kordis PL: Strategy of the dolphin: scoring a win in a chaotic world, New York, 1989, William Morrow.

Lynch-Sauer J: Using a phenomenological research method to study nursing phenomena. In Leininger M, editor: Qualitative research methods in nursing, Orlando, Fla, 1985, Grune & Stratton, Inc.

MacPhail J: Promoting collaboration between education and practice, Nurse Educator 5:19-21, 1976.

MacStravic S: Warfare or partnership; which way for health care? Healthcare Management Rev 15(1):37-45, 1990.

Manthey M: Delivery systems and practice models: a dynamic balance, Nurs Management 22(1):28-30, 1991.

Maraldo PJ and Solomon SB: Nursing's window of opportunity, Image J Nurs Scholarship 19(2):83-86, 1987.

Marlinko MJ and Gardner WL: Learned helplessness: an alternative explanation for performance deficits, Acad Management Rev 7(2):195-204, 1983.

Martin D: The Planetree model hospital project, An example of the patient as partner, Hosp Health Services Adm 35(4):591-601, 1990.

Maslow A: Motivation and personality, New York, 1954, Harper & Row.

Matejski M: Politics, the nurse, and the political process, Nurs Leadership, p 31, March 1979.

Mayo E: Human problems of an industrial civilization, New York, 1933, Macmillan Co.

Mayo E: The social problems of an industrial civilization, Boston, 1945, Harvard Business School.

McDonagh K, editor: Nursing shared governance; restructuring for the future, Atlanta, Ga, 1990, KJ McDonagh & Associates Inc.

McGregor D: The human side of enterprise, New York, 1960, McGraw-Hill Book Co.

McLaughlin C and Kaluzny A: Total quality management in health; making it work, Healthcare Management Rev 15(3):7-14, 1990.

McNeil J: An administrator's view of staff education needs, Nurs Outlook, pp 641-645, October 1978.

Mink O, Shultz J, and Mink B: Developing and managing open organizations, Austin, Tex, 1979, Learning Concepts, Inc.

Mitnick SD and Crumette BD: Hospital nurses as entrepreneurs, Nurs Management 18(11):58-64, 1987.

Moos R: The social climate scales, A user's guide, Palo Alto, Calif, 1987, Consulting Psychologists Press.

Moses E and Roth A: Nursepower, Am J Nurs 79:1745-1758, 1979.

Mowday RT, Steers RM, and Porter LW: The measure of organizational commitment, J Vocational Behav 14:224-247, 1979.

Munhall P: Methodological issues in nursing research: beyond a wax apple, Adv Nurs Sci 8:1-5, 1986.

Munhall P and Oiler C, editors: Epistemology in nursing. In Nursing research: a qualitative perspective, Norwalk, Conn, 1986, Appleton-Century-Crofts.

Muff J: Socialization, sexism, and stereotyping women's issues in nursing, Prospect Heights, Ill, 1988, Waveland Press Inc.

Naisbitt J: Megatrends: ten new directions transforming our lives, New York, 1982, Warner Books, Inc.

Naisbitt J: Reinventing the corporation, New York, 1987, Warner Books, Inc.

National League for Nursing: Characteristics of graduate education in nursing, New York, 1974, The League.

National League for Nursing: Masters education in nursing, 1980, New York, 1980, The League.

National League for Nursing: Some statistics on baccalau-reate and higher degree programs in nursing — 1969, New York, 1970, The League.

Naylor MD and Sherman MB: Nurses for the future: wanted: the best and the brightest, Am J Nurs 87(12):1601-1605, 1987.

Newman MA: Health as expanding consciousness, St Louis, 1986, The CV Mosby Co.

Newcomb T: Social psychology, New York, 1951, Dryden Press.

Noel TM and Devanna MA: The transformational leader, New York, 1986, John Wiley & Sons.

Norman N et al: Statistical package for the social services, New York, 1975, McGraw-Hill Book Co.

Nornhold P: Power: its changing hands and moving your way, Nursing 86 16(1):40-42, 1986.

Orem D: On the scene at St Joseph's Hospital: developing a shared governance model for nursing, Nurs Adm Q, Fall 1982.

Orem D: Nursing: concepts of practice, New York, 1971, McGraw-Hill Co.

Ortiz ME, Gehring P and Sovie MD: Moving to shared governance, Am J Nurs 923-926, July 1987.

Orth C et al: The manager's role as coach and mentor, J Nurs Adm 20(9):11-15, 1990.

Ouchi W: Theory Z: how American business can meet the Japanese challenge, Reading, Mass, 1981, University of Massachusetts Press.

Parse RR: Nursing science: major paradigms, theories, and critiques, Philadelphia, 1987, WB Saunders.

Perry L: Gain sharing plans boost productivity, Modern Healthcare, pp 66, February 12, 1990.

Peters T: Thriving on chaos, New York, 1987, Knopf.

Peters T and Waterman R: In search of excellence: lessons from America's best run companies, New York, 1982, Harper & Row Publishers.

Peterson ME: Motivating staff to participate in decision-making, Nurs Adm Q 7(2):63-68, 1983.

Peterson ME and Allen DG: Shared governance: a strategy for transforming work, Pt. 2, J Nurs Adm 16:11-16, 1986b.

Pinkerton S: Evaluation of shared governance in a nursing department, In Stull M and Pinkerton S, editors: Current strategies for nurse administrators, Rockville, Md, 1988, Aspen Publishers.

Pinkerton SE and Schroeder P: The commitment to excellence: developing a professional nursing staff, Rockville, Md, 1987, Aspen Publishers, Inc.

Porter-O'Grady T: Budgeting for nursing, Supervisor Nurse, pp 35-38, August 1979.

Porter-O'Grady T: Bylaws, an expression of self governance, Perspectives Nurs 1983-85, National League for Nursing, 1983.

Porter-O'Grady T: The nurse administrator's role in cost-effective facilities planning, Nurs Adm Q 2(3):67-73, 1978.

Porter-O'Grady T: A nurse on the board, J Nurs Adm 21(1):40-46, 1991.

Porter-O'Grady T, editor: Nursing staff by-laws and practice privileges, Nurs Adm Q 13(4), 1989.

Porter-O'Grady T: The reorganization of nursing practice, Rockville, Md, 1990, Aspen Publishers.

Porter-O'Grady T: Restructuring the nursing organization for a consumer driven market place, Nurs Adm Q 12(3):60-65, 1988.

Porter-O'Grady T: Shared governance for nursing, Part One: Creating the new organization, AORN J 53(2):458-466, 1991.

Porter-O'Grady T: Shared governance for nursing, Part Two: Putting the organization into action, AORN J 53(3):694-704, 1991.

Porter-O'Grady T: What motivation isn't, Nurs Management, 12(12):23-27, 1982.

Porter-O'Grady T and Finnigan S: Shared governance for nursing: a creative approach to professional accountability, Rockville, Md, 1984, Aspen Systems Corporation.

Porter-O'Grady T and Kanri J: Creating a professional organization for nursing, Nurs Facilitator, pp 3-6, November 1983.

Poulin M: Education for nursing administrator: an epilogue, Nurs Adm Q 3(4):45-51, 1979.

Poulin M: Foreward, Nurs Adm Q 3(4):ix, 1979.

Poulin M: Nursing service: Change or managerial obsolescence, J Nurs Adm, p 40, August 1974.

Poulin M: Study of the structure and functions of the position of nursing service administrator, doctoral dissertation, New York, 1972, Columbia University.

Prescott P and Dennis KE: Power and powerless in hospital nursing departments, J Professional Nurs 1:348-355, 1985.

Reich RB: Who is them? Harvard Bus Rev 69(2):77-88, 1991.

Rimel R: Nurses for the future: searching for excellence, Am J Nurs 87(12):1638-1642, 1987.

Robb CS, editor: Making the connections: essays in feminist social ethics, Boston, 1985, Beacon.

Roberts SJ: Oppressed group behavior: implications for nursing, Adv Nurs Sci 3(2):21-32, 1983.

Robey M: A method of designing a competency based education program to prepare nursing service administrators for complex health care institutions, doctoral dissertation, New York, 1977, Columbia University.

Rogers EM: Diffusion of innovations, ed 3, New York, 1983, The Free Press.

Rose H: What is feminism? In Mitchell J and Oakley, editors: Women's work: women's knowledge, New York, 1986, Pantheon.

Rotkovitch R: A clinical component in education for nursing administration, Nurs Outlook, pp 668-671, October 1979.

Rotkovitch R: The nursing directors' role in money management, J Nurs Adm, pp 13-16, November/December 1981.

Rowland H, editor: The nurses' almanac, Germantown, Md, 1978, Aspen Systems Corp.

Rusch S: Development of a professional managed care nursing model, Unpublished presentation, Center for Nursing Case Management, New England Medical Center, Boston, Mass, April 24, 1987.

Schaeffer M: The knowledge worker, J Nurs Adm, pp 7-9, April 1977.

Scherer P: Hospitals that attract and keep nurses, Am J Nurs 88(1):34-40, 1988.

Schlotfeldt RM: Nursing in the future, Nurs Outlook 29:295-301, 1981.

Schuler R: A role and expectancy perception model of participation in decision-making, Acad Management J 23(2):331-340, 1980.

Senge P: The fifth discipline: The art and practice of the learning organization, New York, 1991, Doubleday/Currency.

Sherwood T: A word about clinical privileging, Nurs Management 22(2):52-54, 1991.

Simpson K: Job satisfaction or dissatisfaction reported by registered nurses, Nurs Adm Q 9:64-73, 1985.

Sims H: Leader structure and subordinate satisfaction for two hospital administrative levels: a path analysis approach, J Applied Psychol 60:194-197, 1975.

Sinentar M: Developing the 21st century mind, New York, 1991, Villard Books.

Slavitt DB et al: Nurses' satisfaction with their work situation, Nurs Res, pp 114-120, March/April 1978.

Sleicher MN: Nursing is not a profession, Nurs Healthcare 2:186-191, 1981.

Sloane R: A guide to health facilities, The American Hospital Association, 1981.

Spitzer R: The nurse in the corporate world, Nurs Management, pp 21-24, April 1981.

Stamps P and Piedmonte E: Nurses and work satisfaction. Ann Arbor, Mich, 1986, Health Administration Press Perspectives.

Standards of nursing practice, Kansas City, Mo, 1973, American Nurses Association.

Stayer R: How I learned to let my workers lead, Harvard Bus Rev 68(6): 66-93, 1990.

Stevens B: Administration of nursing services: a platform for practice, In Administration present and future, New York, 1978, National League for Nursing.

Stevens B: Education in nursing administration, Supervisor Nurse, pp 19-23, March 1977.

Stevens B: Power and politics for the nurse executive, Nurs Health Care, pp 208-212, November 1980.

Stivers C: Why can't a woman be less like a man? J Nurs Adm 21(5):47-51, 1991.

Stogdell R, and Coons A, editors: Leader behavior: its description and measurement, Research Monologue No. 88, Columbus, 1957, Ohio State University, Bureau of Business Research.

Stull MK and Pinkerton SE: Current strategies for nurse administrators, Rockville, Md, 1988, Aspen Publishers, Inc.

Styles MM: On nursing: toward a new endowment, St Louis, 1982, The CV Mosby Co.

Talarczyk G and Milbrandt D: A collaborative effort to facilitate role transition from student to registered nurse practitioner, Nurs Management 19:30-32, 1988.

Taylor F: The principles of scientific management, New York, 1911, Harper & Bros.

Tichey N and Dadevanna MA: The transformational leader, New York, 1990, John Wiley & Sons Inc.

Tiffany C and Cruise P: Discretion and professionalization: a correlational study, Nurs Management 19(2): 72A-72P, 1988.

Toffler A: Powershift, New York, 1990, Bantam Books.

Toffler A: The third wave, New York, 1980, W Morrow & Company, Inc.

Tonges M: Re-designing hospital nursing practice, J Nurs Adm 19(7):31-38, 1989.

Townsend M: Creating a better work environment, J Nurs Adm 21(1):11-14, 1991.

Vanevenhoven R: Job satisfaction for nurses: the theory, the research, the recommendations, unpublished master's thesis, Milwaukee, Wis, 1987, Marquette University.

Vlcek D: Decentralization: What works and what doesn't, J Nurs Strategy 8(2):71-74, 1987.

Vogt J and Murrel K: Empowerment in organizations, San Diego, 1990, University Associates Inc.

Vonsell M, Brief A, and Schuler R: Role conflict and ambiguity: integration of the literature and directions for future research, Hum Rel 34(1):43-71, 1981.

Wade LL: The heateric model, Hum Organ 26:40-46, 1967.

Wandelt M, Pierce P, and Widdowson R: Why nurses leave nursing and what can be done about it, Am J Nurs 81:62-77, 1981.

Waterman R: The renewal factor, New York, 1987, Bantam Books.

Weeks LC and Schneider W: Professional practice: the head nurse sets the climate, Nurs Management 18(6):48A-48H, 1987.

Weins A: Expanding nurse autonomy, J Nurs Adm 20(12):15-22, 1990.

Welsch H and LaVan H: Inter-relationships between organizational commitment and job characteristics, job satisfaction, professional behavior and organizational climate, Hum Rel 24(12):1079-1089, 1981.

Werner J: Joint endeavors: the way to bring service and education together, Nurs Outlook 9:546-550, 1980.

Whetstone W: The nurse administrator: A study in perceptions of competencies needed for management effectiveness, doctoral dissertation, 1977, University of Pittsburgh.

White H: Perceptions of leadership styles by nurses in supervisory positions, J Nurs Adm 2(2):6-10, 1971.

Whitte J: Democracy, authority and alienation in work, Chicago, 1980, The University of Chicago Press.

York C and Fecteau DL: Innovative models for professional nursing practice, Nurs Economics 5(4):6-10, 1987.

Zander K: Comparative models of peer consultation. In Shields JD, editor: Peer consultation in a group context, New York, 1985, Springer Publication Co.

Zuboff S: In the age of the smart machine: the future of work and power, New York, 1984, Basic Books, Inc.

Hospitals Implementing Shared Governance

The hospitals identified in this appendix are in different stages of implementing shared governance. They are listed here not because they are especially recommended but because they have committed their energy and resources to full implementation. These hospitals are but a small sample of those across the country that are implementing shared governance in one of its many forms.

It is estimated that over 1,000 hospitals and health care agencies are in some phase of implementing the partnership models typical of the shared governance concept. As the need to invest the professional worker grows in the workplace, more organizations will adapt new organizational and work models. If a site in your region is creating a worker partnership model or shared governance, contact the people there and begin the networking process of information sharing and relationship building. Those who have been involved in shared governance for some time have found that networking is helpful in building the concept of shared governance and avoiding pitfalls in its implementation.

Inclusion of a hospital in this listing does not indicate willingness to share or participate in information sharing or development assistance. However, in my experience few shared governance settings are unwilling to assist others in implementing the concept. Helping develop the concept is fundamental to the beliefs associated with the concept. Please be aware, however, that some agencies charge for their services and information. It is advisable to clarify this with any agency before asking for information or support.

Albert Einstein Medical Center
York & Tabor Roads
Philadelphia, PA 19141

Allentown Hospital Lehigh Medical Center
1200 South Cedar Crest Blvd.
Allentown, PA 18105

Baptist Medical Center
Taylor at Marian Street
Columbia, SC 29220

Archbishop Bergen Mercy Hospital
7500 Mercy Road
Omaha, NE 68124

Borgess Medical Center
1521 Gull Road
Kalamazoo, MI 49001

The Catherine McAuley Health Center
P.O. Box 1127
Ann Arbor, MI 48106

Children's Hospital Medical Center
Elland & Bethesda Avenues
Cincinnati, OH 45229

Fairbanks Memorial Hospital
1650 Cowles Street
Fairbanks, AK 99701

Franklin Square Hospital
9000 Franklin Square Drive
Baltimore, MD 21237

The Greater Baltimore Medical Center
6701 North Charles Street
Baltimore, MD 21204

Heartland Hospital East
5325 Faraon Street
St. Joseph, MO 64506

Henry Ford Hospital
2799 West Grand Boulevard
Detroit, MI 48202

Hunterdon Medical Center
Route 31
Flemington, NJ 08822

Johns Hopkins Hospital
600 North Wolfe Street
Baltimore, MD   21205

Lac-Rancho Los Amigos Medical Center
7601 East Imperial Highway
Downey, CA   90242

MacNeal Hospital
3249 South Oak Park Avenue
Berwyn, IL   60402

Memorial Hospital at Gulfport
P.O. Box 1810
Gulfport, MS   39502

Mercy Hospital & Medical Center
4077 Fifth Avenue
San Diego, CA   92103

Meridian Park Hospital
P.O. Box 3796
Tualatin, OR   97208

Morristown Memorial Hospital
100 Madison Avenue
Morristown, NJ   07960

Mount Sinai Hospital
500 Blue Hills Avenue
Hartford, CT   06112

North Memorial Medical Center
3300 North Oakdale
Robbinsdale, MN   55422

Providence Medical Center
4805 Northeast Glisan Street
Portland, OR   97213

Rex Hospital
4420 Lake Boone Trail
Raleigh, NC   27607

Richland Memorial Hospital
5 Richland Medical Park
Columbia, SC   29203

Riverview Medical Center
One Riverview Plaza
Red Bank, NJ   07701

Rose Medical Center
3567 East Ninth Street
Denver, CO   80220

Roseville Community Hospital
333 Sunrise Avenue
Roseville, CA   95661

Rush-Presbyterian-St. Luke's Medical Center
700 South Paulina
Chicago, IL   60612

Scottsdale Memorial Hospital
7400 East Osborn Road
Scottsdale, AZ   85251

Sharp Memorial Hospital
7901 Frost Street
San Diego, CA   92123

Sinai Samaritan Medical Center
P.O. Box 04667
Milwaukee, WI   04667

Sioux Valley Hospital
1100 South Euclid Avenue
Sioux Falls, SD   57117

Spohn Hospital
600 Elizabeth Street
Corpus Christi, TX   78404

St. Joseph's Hospital
5665 Peachtree Dunwoody Road
Atlanta, GA   30342

St. Luke's Regional Medical Center
190 East Bannock Street
Boise, ID   83712

St. Luke's Episcopal Hospital
6720 Bertner Avenue
Houston, TX   77030

St. Luke's Hospital
44th and Wornall
Kansas City, MO   64111

St. Luke's Medical Center
2900 West Oklahoma Avenue
Milwaukee, WI   53215

St. Mary's Hospital & Health Center
1601 West St. Mary's Road
Tucson, AZ   85745

St. Michael Hospital
2400 West Villard Avenue
Milwaukee, WI   53209

St. Vincent Hospital
25 Winthrop Street
Worcester, MA   01604

Strong Memorial Hospital of the University of Rochester
601 Elmwood Avenue
Rochester, NY   14642

Suburban Hospital
8600 Old Georgetown Road
Bethesda, MD   20814

University of Maryland Shock Trauma Center
22 South Greene Street
Baltimore, MD   21201

Washoe Medical Center
77 Pringle Way
Reno, NV   89520

Research Instruments

A variety of research instruments is available to those wishing to study implementation strategies and movement toward shared governance. As indicated in this workbook, annual evaluation of progress is advised to assess whether substantive changes have occurred and to assess the progress made toward goal fulfillment.

The instruments included in this appendix have been used extensively in shared governance implementation and have proven valuable to their users. While these are not the only available research tools, they do provide an excellent beginning for the evaluation process and are quite successful in assessing progress. Readers are encouraged to contact the authors of these instruments for information regarding use and evaluation.

In addition to the examples of instruments provided in this appendix, it is recommended that organizations develop individualized tools to assess the kinds of changes important to them relative to implementing shared governance. Some institutions evaluate progress, turnover, vacancy, staff satisfaction, clinical impact, relations with the medical staff and other departments, and a host of other factors important to them. Keeping data as the implementation unfolds is a viable way to evaluate progress and the success of certain strategies for implementing shared governance.

STICHLER COLLABORATIVE BEHAVIOR SCALE (CBS)

The Stichler Collaborative Behavior Scale (CBS), comprised of two parts, was developed to measure respondents' perceptions of collaborative behaviors between the nurse and the physician (Part 1) and between the nurse and the manager (Part 2) in a specific departmental relationship. The CBS was developed using a conceptual framework relating to interactional theory and social theory.

The CBS measures the amount of power balancing, interacting, and interpersonal valuing that occurs in a collaborative relationship. The scale has been used to measure the effect of collaboration on predicting job satisfaction and anticipated turnover. Nurse-physician collaborative behavior and nurse-manager collaborative behavior significantly predicted job satisfaction. Only nurse-manager collaborative behavior significantly predicted anticipated turnover.[1]

The content validity index for the instrument is 0.91. Reliability using Chronbach's alpha is 0.96 for the CBS-1 and 0.98 for the CBS-2. Convergent and discriminant validity were established using the multitrait, multimethod approach.

Further information about the psychometric properties of the Collaborative Behavior Scale and permission to use this instrument in further research can be obtained from the author:

Jaynelle F. Stichler, RN, DNS, CNAA
14322 Blue Sage Road
Poway, CA 92064
(619) 451-0298

---

[1]Stichler JF: The effects of collaboration, organizational climate, and job stress on job satisfaction and anticipated turnover, Ann Arbor, MI, University Microfilms, Inc, 1991.

Nurse-Physician Collaborative Behavior Scale–Part 1

Directions: The purpose of this scale is to determine the extent of collaborative behaviors which generally exist between you and the *physicians* with whom you work. (For each statement check (√) the one box that indicates how often you believe that each behavioral statement occurs.) There are no right or wrong answers. Please answer each item as best you can.

	Rarely 1	Sometimes 2	Often 3	Nearly Always 4
1. We feel free to share ideas with one another.				
2. We acknowledge one another's competence.				
3. We support each other as team members.				
4. We work as partners.				
5. We are committed to working together as a team.				
6. We trust one another.				
7. There is a sharing of expertise and talents between us.				
8. We work as "equals" or "partners" for the accomplishment of some goals.				
9. We work together as a team.				
10. My opinions are listened to.				
11. I feel that my input is truly valued.				
12. We work together as associates.				
13. There is a feeling of mutual regard and respect.				
14. We make an effort to resolve any conflicts which arise to our mutual satisfaction.				
15. We both actively participate in the relationship in order to meet our patient care goals.				
16. We share information openly with one another.				
17. We problem solve together.				
18. We recognize the need to have a sense of "give and take" in the relationship.				
19. We recognize our interdependence with one another in order to meet our goals.				
20. We are committed to the process of working together to meet our goals.				

Nurse-Manager Collaborative Behavior Scale–Part 2

Directions: The purpose of this scale is to determine the extent of collaborative behaviors which generally exist between you and the *managers* with whom you work. (For each statement check (√) the one box that indicates how often you believe that each behavioral statement occurs.) There are no right or wrong answers. Please answer each item as best you can.

	Rarely 1	Sometimes 2	Often 3	Nearly Always 4
1. We feel free to share ideas with one another.				
2. We acknowledge one another.				
3. We support each other as team members.				
4. We work as partners.				
5. We are committed to working together as a team.				
6. We trust one another.				
7. There is a sharing of expertise and talents between us.				
8. We work as "equals" or "partners" for the accomplishment of some goals.				
9. We work together as a team.				
10. My opinions are listened to.				
11. I feel that my input is truly valued.				
12. We work together as associates.				
13. There is a feeling of mutual regard and respect.				
14. We make an effort to resolve any conflicts which arise to our mutual satisfaction.				
15. We both actively participate in the relationship in order to meet our patient care goals.				
16. We share information openly with one another.				
17. We problem solve together.				
18. We recognize the need to have a sense of "give and take" in the relationship.				
19. We recognize our interdependence with one another in order to meet our goals.				
20. We are committed to the process of working together to meet our goals.				

NURSE OPINION QUESTIONNAIRE (NOQ)

The Nurse Opinion Questionnaire (NOQ) was developed and initially tested by Dr. Ruth Ludemann and the Nursing Research Committee at Rose Medical Center, Denver, Colorado.[1] It has since been used by the Scottsdale Memorial Hospital Shared Governance Research Committee annually since 1987 to evaluate changes in nurses' perceptions during the implementation of a shared governance structure.

The NOQ contains five scales to measure staff perceptions of variables believed to be affected by shared governance. Organizational commitment is measured by a scale originally developed by Mowday et al (1979)[2] and is not included in this publication. Commitment to shared governance was developed by the Rose Medical Center Research team, with items similar to the organizational commitment scale. Work environment was adapted by the Rose Medical Center Research team from a scale originally used by Welsch and LaVan (1981)[3] and measures perceptions of staff toward the workplace. The scale was shortened from 42 items to 18 items after a factor analysis. Influence was developed by the investigators and measures the amount of influence staff perceive within the organization. Job satisfaction, developed by the team, measures intrinsic and extrinsic job satisfaction.

Reliability coefficients (Cronbach's alpha) have been consistently acceptable, ranging from 0.74 to 0.95, with the majority being above 0.90 over the years.

Permission to use, scoring instructions, and further information may be obtained by contacting Ruth Ludemann, R.N., Ph.D., at Arizona State University, College of Nursing, Tempe, AZ 85287-2602.

---

[1]Ludemann R and Brown C: Staff perceptions of shared governance, Nurs Admi Q 13(4):49-56, 1989.

[2]Mowday RT, Steers RM, and Porter IW: The measure of organizational commitment, J Voc Behavior 14:224-247, 1979.

[3]Welsch H and LaVan H: Inter-relationships between organizational commitment and job characteristics, job satisfaction, professional behavior and organizational climate, Human Relations 24(12):1079-1089, 1981.

Dear Professional Nurse:

Enclosed is a comprehensive questionnaire designed to obtain nurses' opinions about Shared Governance and your perceptions about the work environment.

We would appreciate your assistance in the completion of this evaluation. The information collected will be used to help us understand what is working well for you, what in the Nursing Division needs attention, and what you would like to see included in future planning. We will be collecting this information approximately once a year, as we refine our shared governance program.

All of this information will be collected and reported anonymously, as group information. You cannot be identified individually. The results, when published, will represent group information.

Your participation is voluntary. Your input is valued and we urge you to complete this questionnaire. The more responses we receive, the better understanding we will have about your opinions and concerns. Please return the completed survey *WITHIN TEN DAYS* to a Shared Governance box in the following locations:

6E Conference Room	2W Conference Room
5E Conference Room	SNF Conference Room
4E/Rehab Conference Room	6th Floor Nursing Office
3EA/Telemetry Conf. Room	SCU Lounge
OB Conference Room	

If you have any questions about the research or your participation, feel free to contact any member of the research committee. The results of this study will be shared with the Nursing Coordinating Council annually. If you wish to obtain a copy of the results, please contact a member of the Shared Governance Research Committee.

Thank you in advance for your participation in this project.

The Shared Governance Research Committee

Lisa Block
Wendy Lyons
Barbara Roberts
Lindsay Thomas
Mary Hays, Administrative Consultant
Ruth Ludeman, Ph.D., Principal Investigator

BACKGROUND INFORMATION

Please complete the following information as it applies to you.

1. Have you completed a research questionnaire to evaluate the Shared Governance structure in previous years?

     _____ 1. Yes
     _____ 2. No

2. What is your age?   _____20-29   _____40-49   _____>60
                                   _____ 30-39   _____50-59

3. What is your sex?   _____1. Male   _____2. Female

Employment Information

4. What shift do you work?

     _____ 1. Days
     _____ 2. Evenings
     _____ 3. Nights

5. Are you currently working:

     _____ 1. 8-hour shifts
     _____ 2. 10-hour shifts
     _____ 3. 12-hour shifts

6. What is the nature of your work?

     _____ 1. Patient care
     _____ 2. Patient care plus some management
     _____ 3. Management only
     _____ 4. Expanded role

7. In which clinical nursing service are you employed? (Check one)

_____ 1. Medical-Surgical/Rehabilitation/Staffing Resources/Skilled
           Nursing Facility
_____ 2. Critical Care/Telemetry
_____ 3. OR/PACU/Special Procedures
_____ 4. Maternal Child Services
_____ 5. Nursing Administration

8. What is your present employment status?

_____ 1. 80-hours per pay period
_____ 2. 72-hours per pay period
_____ 3. 64-hours per pay period
_____ 4. > 48-hours, but < 64-hours per pay period
_____ 5. 48-hours per pay period
_____ 6. < 48-hours per pay period

9. How long have you been employed at Scottsdale Memorial Hospital?

_____ years

10. Approximately how many years have you worked in nursing altogether?

_____ years

11. What type of *basic R.N. education* have you completed?

_____ 1. Associate Degree
_____ 2. B.S.N.
_____ 3. Diploma

12. What is the highest level of education you have completed?

   _____ 1. Associate Degree
   _____ 2. B.S.N.
   _____ 3. Diploma
   _____ 4. Baccalaureate non-nursing
   _____ 5. Master's (nursing)
   _____ 6. Master's (non-nursing) Specialty?_____
   _____ 7. Other (specify)_____

13. Are you currently enrolled in a degree program?

   _____ 1. BSN
   _____ 2. BS - non-nursing
   _____ 3. Master's, nursing
   _____ 4. Master's - non-nursing
   _____ 5. Other

Shared Governance Information - some people have not had the opportunity to participate in Shared Governance. Please answer to the best of your ability.

14. Have you served as a chairperson/chair-elect of a Shared Governance Council/Committee in the last year?

   _____ 1. Yes
   _____ 2. No

15. Have you particpated on Shared Governance Councils/Committees in the last year?

   _____ 1. If yes, how many?_____
   _____ 2. No

16. In the last year, how often have you participated in Shared Governance decision making?

   _____ 1. Frequently
   _____ 2. Some
   _____ 3. Seldom
   _____ 4. Never

17. What do you personally see as the main benefit of having Shared Governance?

_____
_____
_____
_____
_____
_____
_____
_____
_____

18. What do you see as the major disappointment and/or problem of Shared Governance?

_____
_____
_____
_____
_____
_____
_____
_____
_____

19. What suggestions do you have for improvement?

_____
_____
_____
_____
_____
_____
_____
_____
_____

Did you work in this hospital prior to the beginning of shared governance (1986)?

_____ 1. Yes   _____ 2. No

NURSING COMMITTEES/COUNCILS AND SHARED GOVERNANCE

Listed below are similar statements that represent possible feelings individuals may have about Shared Governance. Again, please indicate the degree of *your* agreement or disagreement with each statement by circling one of the seven alternatives.

1 = Strongly Disagree (SD)   5 = Mildly Agree (MA)
2 = Disagree (D)   6 = Agree (A)
3 = Mildly Disagree (MD)   7 = Strongly Agree (SA)
4 = No Opinion (NO)

	SD	D	MD	NO	MA	A	SA
1. I am not really very familiar with the structure and functions of our nursing councils and committees.	1	2	3	4	5	6	7
2. I am willing to put in a great deal of effort beyond that normally expected in order for our nursing councils and committees to be successful.	1	2	3	4	5	6	7
3. I talk up shared goverance to my friends as a great way for staff to participate in decision-making which affects their job.	1	2	3	4	5	6	7
4. I feel very little loyalty to the shared goverance councils.	1	2	3	4	5	6	7
5. The physicians at this hospital understand the shared governance program.	1	2	3	4	5	6	7

	SD	D	MD	NO	MA	A	SA
6. Nursing councils and committees really inspire the very best in me in the way of job performance.	1	2	3	4	5	6	7
7. From what I've heard or observed, patient feelings about the quality of nursing care improved with shared governance.	1	2	3	4	5	6	7
8. From what I've heard or observed, nurse-physician relationships have not improved with shared governance.	1	2	3	4	5	6	7
9. For me, shared governance is the best of all possible ways to structure the nursing division.	1	2	3	4	5	6	7
10. From what I've heard or observed, the quality of nursing care has not improved since shared governance started.	1	2	3	4	5	6	7
11. I really do not care about the fate of shared governance.	1	2	3	4	5	6	7
12. Shared governance has turned out to benefit management more than it benefits employees.	1	2	3	4	5	6	7

	SD	D	MD	NO	MA	A	SA
13. The physicians at this hospital are not supportive of the shared governance program.	1	2	3	4	5	6	7
14. From what I've heard or observed, the comprehansiveness and continuity of nursing care have not improved with the shared governance program.	1	2	3	4	5	6	7

Please indicate the degree of *your* agreement or disagreement with each statement by circling one of the six alternatives.

1 = Strongly Disagree (SD)   4 = Mildly Agree (MA)
2 = Disagree (D)   5 = Agree (A)
3 = Mildly Disagree (MD)   6 = Strongly Agree (SA)

	SD	D	MD	MA	A	SA
1. My superior rarely seeks out my input before decisions are made.	1	2	3	4	5	6
2. There are continuing unrealistic pressures from nursing administration for innovation in the way we carry out our activities.	1	2	3	4	5	6
3. I am often unable to influence my immediate supervisor's decisions and actions that affect me.	1	2	3	4	5	6
4. People are proud of being associated with this hospital.	1	2	3	4	5	6
5. If I make a suggestion in decision making, it is usually considered.	1	2	3	4	5	6

	SD	D	MD	MA	A	SA

6. There is a strong desire among personnel in this hospital to keep abreast of innovations that are occurring in the health care area.

     1   2   3   4   5   6

7. We are encouraged to speak our minds, even if it means disagreeing with our superiors.

     1   2   3   4   5   6

8. There is a lot of support from co-workers during innovation attempts.

     1   2   3   4   5   6

9. I rarely have to do things on the job that are against my better judgement.

     1   2   3   4   5   6

10. As far as I can see, there isn't very much personal loyalty to this hospital by the people who work here.

     1   2   3   4   5   6

11. There is a strong commitment among personnel in this hospital to working through the problems that accompany change and innovation.

     1   2   3   4   5   6

12. There is a lot of cooperation among the different departments in this hospital in trying to implement-utilize innovations into our ongoing activities.

     1   2   3   4   5   6

	SD	D	MD	MA	A	SA
13. I have too heavy a work load, one that I cannot finish during an ordinary work day.	1	2	3	4	5	6
14. It is easy to get necessary information for decision making.	1	2	3	4	5	6
15. My supervisor in this hospital does make an effort to talk with me about my career aspirations.	1	2	3	4	5	6
16. I have little opportunity to participate in innovative changes.	1	2	3	4	5	6
17. The amount of work I routinely have to do does not interfere with how well it gets done.	1	2	3	4	5	6
18. I have too much responsibility delegated to me by my supervisors.	1	2	3	4	5	6

INFLUENCE

Please indicate the degree of *your* agreement or disagreement with each statement by circling one of the six alternatives.

1 = No Influence (N)   4 = Moderate Influence (M)
2 = Little Influence (L)   5 = Great Influence (G)
3 = Some Influence (S)   6 = No Opinion/Don't Know (NO)

How much influence does
the staff have:

	N	L	S	M	G	NO
1. To influence changes in nursing services.	1	2	3	4	5	6
2. With hospital administration.	1	2	3	4	5	6
3. With nursing administration.	1	2	3	4	5	6
4. To make decisions on issues that affect nursing.	1	2	3	4	5	6
5. To influence changes in policy and procedure.	1	2	3	4	5	6
6. To influence changes in personnel policies.	1	2	3	4	5	6
7. To propose new ideas for consideration.	1	2	3	4	5	6
8. To influence the quality of nursing.	1	2	3	4	5	6

Please indicate the degree of *your* agreement or disagreement with each statement by circling one of the six alternatives.

1 = Very Dissatisfied (VD)   4 = Barely Satisfied (BS)
2 = Dissatisfied (D)   5 = Satisfied (S)
3 = A Little Dissatisfied (LD)   6 = Very Satisfied (VS)

How satisfied are you with:	VD	D	LD	BS	S	VS
1. The feeling of self-esteem or self-respect a person gets from being in your job?	1	2	3	4	5	6
2. The opportunities for personal growth and career development in your job?	1	2	3	4	5	6
3. The prestige of your job inside the hospital (that is, the regard received from others in the hospital)?	1	2	3	4	5	6
4. The opportunity for independent thought and action in your job?	1	2	3	4	5	6
5. The pay for your job?	1	2	3	4	5	6
6. The feeling of worthwhile accomplishment in your job?	1	2	3	4	5	6
7. The opportunity in your job for participation in the determination of methods, procedures, and goals?	1	2	3	4	5	6

	VD	D	LD	BS	S	VS
8. The opportunity for clinical promotion?	1	2	3	4	5	6
9. The opportunity for managerial promotion?	1	2	3	4	5	6
10. The amount of respect and fair treatment I receive from your supervisor?	1	2	3	4	5	6
11. The feeling of being informed about what's happening in the nursing division?	1	2	3	4	5	6
12. The prestige of your job outside the hospital (that is, the regard received from others not in the hospital)?	1	2	3	4	5	6
13. Your work schedule and hours?	1	2	3	4	5	6

There may be feelings or ideas that you wish to express, about your work or about Shared Governance which are not addressed in this questionnaire. Please feel free to share these thoughts in the space below.

RESEARCH INSTRUMENT BY DAVID ALLEN

This instrument has been adjusted and individualized in a number of settings where it has been applied. To ensure that any individualization does not invalidate the instrument, it is recommended that the instrument's author be contacted directly regarding use and adaptation. For this reason, a sample of the instrument is not provided in this appendix but a description of it follows.

The variables comprising the instrument include the following: (1) participation in decision making (3 scales); (2) job discretion/difficulty (a measure of how difficult one's daily work is and the degree of discretion one has in job-related decisions); (3) internal motivation; (4) role conflict; (5) organizational commitment and; (6) job satisfaction.

Scales addressing variables can be deleted, depending on the design of the study. The instrument can be used to measure the degree of participation and correlational or causal relationships between participation and other variables (e.g., satisfaction).

The instrument is based on a theoretical model and is composed of well-established scales from prior research and ones developed by the author. Reliability and validity is excellent for all scales. The tool has been used in over 12 organizations with approximately 3,000 nurses comprising the data base. An analysis and/or comparison data from matched organizations may be procured from the author (at cost). There is no charge for use of this instrument but an agreement with other authors requires sharing data and codebooks.

Contact David Allen, RN, PhD, FAAN at (206) 543-3112 for further information.

Sample Questionnaires

Development is perhaps the single most important element of shared governance implementation. Entirely new roles and behaviors will have to emerge from the staff if the process is to be successful. Not all staff are ready or prepared for many of the new accountabilities and attendant roles and authorities that accompany the move to shared governance. A host of developmental activities will need to emerge from the organization if nurses are to be successful in their new staff leadership roles.

Each organization should devise instruments that help the individual assess his or her behavior, role, and progress in moving toward new expectations and responsibilities. These instruments do not have to be sophisticated. They do need to be direct and helpful to the participant in exploring specific issues and circumstances related to the role responsibility and the skill level of the individual.

Following are some brief and directed samples of questionnaires that can be helpful to staff and management as they explore the impact of implementing shared governance. These questionnaires can be duplicated, if helpful, and used in whatever way facilitates development. They are most useful to those in leadership roles but can be used by staff at any organizational level. The data generated should be helpful to the individual in discovering and/or developing leadership skills. They may also serve as a guide for the formulation of questionnaires representing specified interests in individual organizations.

READINESS FOR COUNCIL CHAIR QUESTIONNAIRE

Completion of this questionnaire will help the potential group leader understand what needs and strengths are involved in the group leader role. Developmental activities can then be adjusted to the needs of the role and the skills of the individual.

Answer the following based on your understanding of yourself as a group leader:

Have I had experience as a group leader before?
If yes:

My greatest strength was:

My greatest weakness was:

I wish I had done better at:

My greatest fear was:

My greatest satisfaction was:

I would say my greatest group skills are:
1.

2.

3.

My greatest fear is:

I think I can do well at:
1.

2.

My role model is:

What skills does this person exemplify?

What skill would I most like to emulate?

What is my greatest skill?

Why do I want a leadership role?

What does this role demand?
1.

2.

3.

4.

5.

What skill development do I most need to undertake?

What resources are available to me?

Group facilitation skills

How strong is my skill level in the following areas of group leadership? (Rate the skills on a scale of one to five, one being the lowest level of skill and five being the highest.)

_____ Consensus seeking
_____ Conflict resolution
_____ Group facilitating
_____ Decision making
_____ Problem solving
_____ Rules of conduct
_____ Goal focusing
_____ Solution seeking
_____ Obtaining support and resources

What personal developmental agenda can I create based on this assessment of my skills?
1.

2.

3.

4.

How will I get these needs met?

Where?

From whom?

Time frame?

CONFLICT MANAGEMENT QUESTIONNAIRE

Conflict almost always engenders fear and uncertainty. The good leader can manage conflict situations and use conflict to improve dialogue and move to newer levels of interaction. This instrument helps determine individual response to conflict and identify barriers to good management.

When people I work with have conflict I usually:

_____ Intervene
_____ Avoid
_____ Support
_____ Take sides

When someone I care for acts out toward me I feel:

_____ Hostile
_____ Afraid
_____ Concerned
_____ Assertive
_____ Other _____

If I am attacked in a meeting, I usually:

_____ Ignore it
_____ Fight
_____ Understand
_____ Become quiet and passive
_____ Cry
_____ Other _____

When I see conflict not directed toward me I:

_____ Mediate
_____ Watch
_____ Take sides
_____ Get away
_____ Tell others

When I look at the above responses I find that I most often respond to conflict by:

I wish I could do the following in a conflict situation:
1.

2.

3.

To be successful in handling conflict I would have to make the following personal changes:
1.

2.

3.

My personal response to a tense situation that could result in conflict is to:

     _____ Use humor
     _____ Deflect to another issue
     _____ Out talk the situation
     _____ Problem solve
     _____ Disappear

My specific developmental plan for dealing with conflict is:

    1.

    2.

    3.

Resources available for me to learn to deal with conflict are:

    1.

    2.

    3.

Specific learning objectives for me are:

    1.

    2.

    3.

Time frame for learning to deal with conflict is:

Outcomes I would like to see in my ability to deal with conflict are:

    1.

    2.

TEAM-BUILDING QUESTIONNAIRE

Virtually all shared governance leadership involves teams. The whole process of working in shared governance organizations is team based. Developing team-building skills is challenging but possible when one knows what must be done and how to go about doing it. This questionnaire explores the efforts directed at team building and the individual skills essential to it.

Goals

Does each member of the group know why he or she is here?

Why does the group exist? What are its purposes?

    1.

    2.

    3.

    4.

5.

What is the group's agenda? What are its goals?

Membership

Are all the members present?

Do they want to be here?

Has there been time for group socialization?

What has been done to encourage group socialization?
1.

2.

3.

Is there a role for all the members of the group?

Are the group expectations enumerated?

_____ Purpose
_____ Time
_____ Expectations
_____ Behaviors
_____ Commitments

Are there consultants and/or advisers available to the group? Is their role clear?

Meeting preparation

Are the following items addressed in meeting preparation?

_____ Agenda
_____ Meeting time
_____ Role expectation of members
_____ Decisions expected

Does the chairperson anticipate discussion? Conflict? The need for information or other resources?

What priorities have been established for the meeting agenda?
1.

2.

3.

4.

Dysfunctional behaviors

Has the leader anticipated the behaviors of the following characters?

- _____ Saboteur
- _____ Sniper
- _____ Shadow chairperson
- _____ Denier of any knowledge
- _____ Terminally quiet member
- _____ Group dominator
- _____ Side tracker
- _____ Permanently safe (no risker)
- _____ Always agree (no disagreement)
- _____ Forever wrong (nothing is right)
- _____ Attention seeker

Constructive interventions

-Translate issues into clear problem statements or opportunities
-Focus the group on the issues at hand
-Monitor group involvement in discussion
-Use strategies for clarification (e.g., pros and cons, critical path, objective setting)
-Move group to decision making and consensus
-Assess level of group energy
-Enumerate group accomplishments

• • •

The team builder is aware of the needs of the team and adjusts the focus to address the issues that facilitate group development. Questions related to successful assessment of team-building needs are:

Are there growing numbers of dysfunctional behaviors?

Are people increasingly disruptive?

Do goals get sidetracked for personal agendas?

Has any socialization been planned for the group?

Does the group take time to celebrate its accomplishments?

Does the chairperson have support and advice and council from an experienced and successful group leader?

Sample Accountabilities, Goals, and Timelines

A sample set of accountabilities, goals, and timelines is included in this appendix to serve as a guide for those setting up an implementation plan for developing shared governance. It is recommended that the reader not replicate this set of guides since they reflect the needs of an individual hospital culture and may not reflect the values and culture of the reader's organization. The specific concerns of the environment must always be incorporated into the planning process. Careful consideration of the strengths and needs of the individual organization must always precede the development of an implementation plan.

The process of planning implementation of shared governance usually falls to the steering group. Assessment of readiness for implementing shared governance and an understanding of the changes implied should be the first step. This assessment will help determine the specific cultural and organizational needs of the individual setting and provide a baseline for planning implementation.

Timelines are helpful in both planning and evaluation processes. Every step or element of shared governance implementation should have an attached set of time parameters. There is so much interdependence in implementing the various components of shared governance that time values become vital to success. They serve as an excellent tool for measuring progress.

MORRISTOWN MEMORIAL HOSPITAL
Morristown, New Jersey

The accountability process

A critical element of the shared governance process is the establishment of council accountabilities and a discussion of potential cooperation zones. Cooperation zones relate to those issues having components that impact more than one council. They require cooperation of multiple councils for problem solving to occur. Final decision-making authority must be assigned to one council. The identi-

fication of overlapping areas compels the council members to discuss the potential issues within the executive council framework. Some of these issues will be highly sensitive and emotionally charged. The environment for discussion becomes crucial to an open and honest exchange of information so that true cooperation can be achieved.

The use of an off-site executive council retreat in a setting conducive to teamwork can facilitate this process. Using a consultant as a facilitator allows the chief nursing officer to participate and experience the transitional phase of this power shift without needing to expend time and energy on directing the group. This approach also provides the executive council with guidance when the goal of assigning accountabilities based on function becomes clouded by historical data (we need to continue to do it that way until we are comfortable with the shift of accountability to a new group) with the philosophical and cultural shift to shared governance (we must trust that the people who are affected will assume the accountability for this issue and must therefore allow them to).

The executive council can assign final authority for decision making to one individual council only when a discussion of all the facets of an accountability are reviewed. Grids can be helpful in identifying both the accountabilities of the councils and the areas requiring cooperation based on individual council accountabilities (Figure E-1). The task of developing such a grid can be accomplished during the executive retreat and should be referred to as the executive council deliberates what council should have final authority to decide certain questionable issues. It can also be referred to when constructing a 5-year timeline for council work.

The organization's mission and goals must be carefully considered along with council accountabilities in establishing a timeline for the shared governance process (Figure 2). This ensures that the nursing division is consistent with the directions set by the Board of Trustees and the presi-

Accountable Council	Issue	Practice
Practice	Conceptual Framework	Decide/Define-X
	Standards/Practice	Decide/Define-X
	Performance Standards	Decide/Define-X
	Position Descriptions-*	Decide/Define-X
	Clinical Ladder - *	Decide/Define-X

Accountable Council	Issue	QI
Quality Improvement (QI)	Plan	Define-X
	Priorities	Define-X
	Unit-Based Activities	Control-X
	Performance Evals-*	Clinical-X
	Clinical Ladder - *	Measure-X
	Credentialing &	Measure-X
	Privileging (Provisional	
	Prioritizing)	
	Research - *	Measure-X

Accountable Council	Issue	Management
Management	Resources - *	Staffing-X
	Human	Scheduling-X
		FTE's-X
		Mix Staff (NHPD)-X
		Ratio-X
	Fiscal	Economics-X
		Budget-X
		Allocation-X
		Capital-X
	Materials - *	Supplies/Equipt-X
		Medical/Clinical
		Support-X
	Support - *	Relation-X
		Counsel-X
		Discipline-X
		Environment-X
		Motivation-X
		Context-X
	Systems	Integrate-X
		Coordinate-X
		Facilitate-X
		Operations-X
		Interdepartmental Fit:Intra-,
		Inter-,SG Unit-X

Accountable Council	Issue	Education
Education	Orientation	Define Program-X
	Educational Program - *	Decide/Define-X
	Unit-Based Education	Decide/Define-X
	Communication	Control-X
	Quarterly Staff Meetings	Decide/Define-X
	School Rotations	Control-X

Key { } =Support Function	Area of accountability that requires the support of another council for accomplishing the goals within that area.	* = Cooperation Zones	Accountabilities that can result in a conflictual relationship if the councils do not cooperate during the problem-solving process.

FIGURE E-1
Accountability grid

QI	Education	Management	Administration
{Measure} {Measure} {Evaluate} {Measure}		{Enforcement} {Management Position Description-X} {Resource Enforcement} {Evaluate} Fiscal	{X} {HR Format} Integrate Fiscally-X

Practice	Education	Management	Administration
{Decide/Define} {Decide/Define} {Decide/Define}	{Orientation} {Orientation}	Resource Control-X Measure Resources-X {Measure-X} Measure/Control-X	{Institution} Human Resource-X Role Conflict:IRB-X Department Fiscal-X

Practice	QI	Education	Administration
{Advise} Standards-X Model of Care-X {Advise} {Advise Products} {Advise} {Clinical Advise} {Fiscal Advise} Performance Standards	{Advise} {Measure/Control}	{Advise}	Fiscal-X Negotiate-X Cuts/Adjustments-X {Advise/Consent}

QI	Practice	Management	Administration
{Measure}	Define Criteria-X	Resource-X Control/Resource-X	Resource Allocation-X {Support Department Obligations}

X = Area of Ownership	Council that has the right to a specific accountability. This can assist the Executive Council in assigning issues to the correct council for decision-making when a conflict exists.

Timeline Year 1 & 2	Accountabilities	June	July	August	September	December	January
Practice Council	Establish Standards of Practice: Generic & Unit-based Do template for Career Advancement Program: Parameters, Format, Approval Mechanism, etc. Define Key Indicators Incorporate Above into Ladder Develop & Implement Evaluation for Above	Theory — Review Material on Theory Based Practice	Evaluate — Nursing Theorists Decide on Four	Define —— Framework & Norms of Nurses at MMH	Select Theory to be Basis of Care at MMH-Complete Plan 1st Quarterly Staff Mtg	——→	Disperse information Re: Theory-I. King Completed via below Complete

Management Council	Incorporate Facilitation rather than Directing Staff into Management Skills/Style
	Implement/Modify Systems to Exemplify Responsible Use of Resources: Human, Material, Fiscal
	Represent MMH Mission & Goals as Councils Deliberate Decisions
	Define Process that Relates QI Council Re:Compliance/Discipline to Management Council
	Establish Systems for:
	  Role Clarification
	  Credentialing & Priviledging
	  Performance Criteria/Definition
		Define —— Accountabilities of all Members: Sr. V.P. Nursing, Directors A.D.'s			————————→	Complete	Establish Mechanism for mentoring A.D.'s

Quality Improvement Council	Link MMH Mission & Goals to QI Priorities Create Design Format for Performance Appraisals, ie: Tools, Timing, Paper, Appeals, Eval., etc. Assess & Refine Career Ladder: Access, Criteria, & Reward System Develop Priviledging System: Entry, Review, Process & Types of Approval Plan & Develop Research Council						
Education Council	Link Orientation w/Practice Council Criteria Set 2-4 Priorities/year Based on QI Data, MMH Mission & Goals, & Identified Staff Needs Fulfill Required Classes: JCAHO, D.O.H., CPR, etc. Define Roles: eg. CNS's, CN III's Establish & Evaluate Mechanisms for Communication						

FIGURE E-2
Six-year timeline

February	March	April	May	June	July	September	October	December
Define Generic Practice Standards ———————→				Complete				
				Format Form Unit-Based Practice Standards ———————→			Complete	
						Implement Nursing Process, Documentation, Assessment, etc ————→		Complete
Plan 2nd-Quarterly Staff Mtg Topic: Unit-Based Shared Governance ————→			Complete	——————→	Evaluate Mechanism Continue or Modify	——————→		Define RN Account-abilities ——→
		Begin Phase I A.D. Support Group ————→			——————→	Start Phase II Group ——————→		——→
		Managers-HR Development Program for Phase II A.D.'s ————→			Develop 1992 Budget ————→		Complete	Establish Mechanism for resolution of Conflicts between Councils ——→
		Implement Staffing w/Medicus ————→		————→	Evaluate-Staffing w/Medicus ————→		Continue-Staffing w/Medicus ————→	
	Set Priorities: Approval Monitoring Eval Corrective Actions ————→			Complete ————→		Complete		——→
			Plan 3rd-Quarterly Staff Mtg Topic: Change		Develop Corrective Action Plan ——→			
		Develop Communication Vehicle	Complete →	Develop Criteria for Confirming Attendance at Programs			Complete	——→
			Attend Team Bldg Day-Complete			Plan & Format Communication Between Councils ————→		

Continued.

Timeline Year 3 & 4	January	March	May	June	July	September	October
Practice Council	Nursing Process w/ I. King-Complete Formalize ——————————————————→ Position Descriptions				Revise —————— Clinical Ladder Complete——		
Management Council	>Phase I Group-Complete Begin Phase III —— Support Group Link Position Descriptions w/ Disciplinary Criteria Performance —— Based Position Descriptions	Establish Guidelines for Link w/ QI Council Re: Discipline ——————————→			Develop —————————————→ Complete 1993 Budget Complete		Complete
Quality Improvement Council	Corrective Action Plan-Complete Review Research Process eg. Submission of —————————————→ Proposals, Actions, Reports	Collaborate w/Managers Re:Discipline Design Peer —— Review/Appeal Process		Complete			
Education Council	Communication ————————————————→ Complete ———————————————→ Evaluate Vehicle Between Councils-Complete Professional Staff Meeting-Complete		Develop —— Process for Staff Mtgs. 3x's/year: 1 Annual & 2 Prof.	Plan Prof. ——————→ Complete Staff Mtg.			

FIGURE E-2—cont'd
Six-year timeline

December	January	May	June	July	September	October	December
⟶	Complete						
⟶			⟶	Evaluate Position Description & Modify Where Appropriate			
⟶Complete	Perform-ance Based Review Linked w/QI		Educating HR Dept. Re: Cred-entialing & Priv-ileging	Develop ⟶ 1994 Budget		Complete	
⟶ Complete	Design ⟶ Career Ladder (Appli-cation, Approv-al, & Cont.)		Credentialing Entry (Review Process & Approval)		Evaluate ⟶ Peer Review Process	⟶ ⟶	Complete Complete ⟶
⟶Complete Learn to Manage Conf Budget Plan Prof ⟶ Meeting	Manage Conf. Budget & Review Monthly ⟶	Complete		Plan ⟶ Prof. Staff Meeting	Assess ⟶ Orientation Process Complete		⟶

Continued.

Timeline Year 5 & 6	January	February	May	June	July	September	October
Practice Council					Evaluate Position Descriptions & Modify if Needed		
Management Council	HR Training Credentialing & Privileging	———————————————→		Complete	Develop 1995 Budget ———————→		Complete
Quality Improvement Council	Credentialing Process (cont.)	———————————————→		Complete			
Education Council	Assess Orientation Process-Complete	Plan ———→ Annual Staff Meeting	Complete		Plan ———→ Prof. Staff Meeting	Complete	Plan Prof. Staff Meeting
	Format Orientation Process ————————————————————————————————→					Evaluate Orientation Process & Modify Complete	
	Examine Educational Programs & Set Standards ———————————————→					Complete	
	Prof. Staff Mtg.-Complete						

FIGURE E-2—cont'd
Six-year timeline

dent of the hospital. Additionally, the discussion of mission and goals should spark a contributory process from the bottom up. Assuring communication flows in all directions is an essential piece of strategic planning for nursing and the organization. The nurse is undoubtedly the individual most likely to hear what the patients' and community members' perceptions of missing services are and what services are rendered well.

In the final analysis, the shared governance process will be evaluated based on the ability of the nursing leaders to plan for, support, and live the power shift that these discussions are aimed at facilitating. Careful consideration of this aspect of the process cannot be overstated in terms of its importance. Staff nurses and managers alike will be carefully assessing to see if the assignment of accountability ownership is consistent with the philosophical shift to shared governance. The use of these tools and strategies can assist in achieving a successful evaluation of the shift to nursing professionalism in today's health care environ-

ment. This cultural change will establish a strong support base for nurses and the organization if allowed to flourish. It is up to each nurse to support this process from whatever vantage point she or he has within an organization. Support is there for nurses.

This material is reprinted with permission from Morristown Memorial Hospital, Morristown, New Jersey. The members who deserve recognition for their role in the development and submission of this material are:

Jean M. McMahon, Sr. V.P. for Nursing
  Chairperson, Executive Council

Trish Baxter, Staff Nurse
  Chairperson, Education Council

Gloria Chappelle, Unit Educator/Staff Nurse
  Chairperson, Practice Council

Nicole Goldstein, Unit Supervisor/Staff Nurse
  Chairperson, Coordinating Council

January	February	May	June	July	September	October
Evaluate Career Ladder & Modify if Needed				Evaluate Position Descriptions & Modify if Needed		
				Develop 1995 Budget ————————→		Complete
——→Complete	Plan ————→ Annual Staff Meeting	Complete		Plan ————→ Prof. Staff Meeting	Complete	Plan ————→ Prof. Staff Meeting

Donna Ilardi, Unit Supervisor/Staff Nurse
Chairperson, Quality Improvement Council

Trish O'Keefe, Administrative Director
Chairperson, Management Council

Bonnie Magliaro, Project Director
Nursing Shared Governance

MORRISTOWN MEMORIAL HOSPITAL
Mission statement

The mission of Morristown Memorial Hospital is to anticipate and respond to the health care needs of the people it serves. In this capacity, Morristown Memorial, as a community hospital and regional referral center, will strive to provide:

1. A comprehensive range of medical and health services of high quality, delivered in the most appropriate environment;

2. A skilled staff working as a team dedicated to the highest attainable standards of health care;

3. An environment in which all patients will be treated with the utmost compassion and respect;

4. Personnel, facilities, and equipment to fulfill these commitments;

5. Training and continuing education for professional and allied health personnel; and,

6. Resources for research and development and for the application of advanced techniques in the health sciences.

This mission will be pursued consistent with responsible fiscal practices and regulatory guidelines.

MORRISTOWN MEMORIAL HOSPITAL
Major goals

1. Recognize and respond to the expectations of the people we serve in everything we do.

2. Enhance our position as the preferred health care provider in Northwest New Jersey.
   2a. Excel as a provider of community and primary care services.
   2b. Continue to grow as the referral center for Northwest New Jersey.
   2c. Become a leading ambulatory care provider.
3. Maintain and support the hospital's medical staff.
4. Maintain an environment conducive to employee satisfaction, retention, and recruitment.
5. Pursue continuous quality improvement.
6. Focus everyone at the Hospital on personal, caring health care service delivery.
7. Recognize and respond effectively to changes in the health care environment.
8. Conduct all activities in a cost-effective manner to assure the continued financial viability of the Hospital.
9. Continuously work to earn the trust and support of the Hospital's publics.

Sample Bylaws

The bylaws presented in this appendix are a representative sample only and are not to be exactly replicated in other organizations. As with other components of implementation, bylaws represent the unique culture of the organization they represent. Each setting will have unique characteristics that influence the design of its shared governance model and thus the bylaws that articulate it.

Bylaws are generally the "last act" of the implementation process. They reflect the sum of the organizational model of shared governance. They serve as an information tool for all who seek to know how the organization operates and how it affects their roles. These bylaws should be descriptive of all the elements of the organization and a solid representation of how it works. The individual reader should be able to discern from the bylaws the functional characteristics of the shared governance process and how to access it and work within its parameters. The bylaws should be clear and well organized, building an understanding of the operation of shared governance as the reader moves through them. Lastly, they should be complete and act as a guide for action by anyone having reference to them.

The following is reprinted with permission from Children's Hospital Medical Center, Cincinnati. The members of the Nursing Executive Council, Division of Nursing who deserve recognition for their role in the development and submission of this material are:

Dorine R. Seaquist, RN

Joann Bailey, RN

Melissa Catania, RN

Pamela J. Morgan, RN

Patricia Lee Messmer, RN

Terri Thrasher, RN

BYLAWS OF CHILDREN'S HOSPITAL MEDICAL CENTER

I. PREAMBLE

The Division of Nursing has instituted the following articles to delineate the responsibility and authority of shared governance within the Division of Nursing, to describe professional nursing and to insure a high level of professional performance by all nursing practitioners authorized to practice as identified in these articles in Children's Hospital Medical Center consistent with the mandates of the Board of Trustees.

Section 1 Philosophy

Nursing is an essential service within Children's Hospital Medical Center for the promotion of the institution's three-fold mission of patient care, education and research.

The Division of Nursing affirms the institution's values of excellence, integrity, and innovation. Every child and family has the right to attain their highest potential whether that be an optimum state of health or a supported, dignified, peaceful death. The goal of nursing is to restore and/or promote the child's and the family's level of health and well-being. The Division of Nursing has adopted the conceptual model articulated by Martha Rogers as a foundational framework for nursing.

The Division of Nursing supports a system that recognizes the shared accountability and responsibility of the decision making process. Finally, as a developing national center for pediatric nursing expertise, the Division of Nursing believes in the responsibility of all nurses at Children's Hospital Medical Center to provide local, state and national leadership in professional pediatric nursing practice.

Section 2 Purposes

The purposes of the Division of Nursing Services are to:
A. Provide quality 24 hour family centered care to all patients and families at Children's Hospital Medical Center.
B. Provide comprehensive, quality patient/family care in collaboration with other health care professionals.
C. Provide an environment that supports shared governance.
D. Provide an environment that supports the growth of the professional nurse and the nursing profession.
E. Participate in development of systems that assist with the advancement of health care programs at Children's Hospital Medical Center and within the community.
F. Provide local, state and national leadership in professional pediatric nursing practice.

Section 3 Critical objectives

A. To provide expert, individualized nursing care through the use of the nursing process within the Rogerian framework.
B. To provide every patient and family with an identified professional nurse who assumes 24 hour accountability for the coordination of that patient and family's nursing care beginning with an admission assessment and continuing through to discharge.
C. To support a system of comprehensive health care provided in collaboration with the patient and family and all other health care providers.
D. To promote ongoing development of patient education systems in the hospital and the community.
E. To promote a professional climate that supports educational opportunities for professional nurses, students and other health care professionals.
F. To ensure optimal patient care through continuous monitoring and evaluation of patient care outcomes and nursing practice.
G. To provide qualified professional nursing staff through an ongoing credentialing and privileging process that incorporates peer evaluation.
H. To provide an environment that promotes, enhances, and supports all aspects of nursing research—generation, dissemination and utilization.
I. To ensure the most effective use of resources, both human and material, within a framework of financial responsibility resulting in optimum patient care.
J. To ensure an environment which enhances the retention and recruitment of qualified nurses.
K. To integrate the nursing profession and the nursing organization through a system of shared accountability and responsibility in the decision making process between all levels of nursing.
L. To participate in the planning process of Children's Hospital Medical Center.

II. ROLE OF THE PROFESSIONAL NURSE

Consistent with the Ohio Nurse Practice Act and the rules and regulations of the Ohio State Board of Nursing, the professional registered nurse (hereinafter referred to as professional nurse) assumes accountability for the delivery of nursing care within the institution. The professional nurse provides care requiring specialized knowledge, judgment, and skill derived from principles of biological, physical, behavioral, social, and nursing sciences. The professional nurse prescribes the nursing care for the patient and educates, administers, supervises, delegates tasks and evaluates nursing practice as it relates to the identified health care needs of the patient. The professional nurse defines and manages the organized delivery of patient care nursing services through contributions to nursing governance councils, committees, and task forces, Medical/Dental Staff committees, and patient-care-related hospital committees. Each professional nurse is accountable to the patient and the nursing organization for the care rendered to the patient. The Board of Trustees through the institutions organizational structure, expects the accountable execution of the nursing professional's role in the delivery of nursing care at CHMC.

III. SERVICES OF NURSING

Registered nurses, in collaboration with other disciplines, coordinate the plan of care of every child/family. Registered nurses prescribe the nursing care of every child/family. Registered nurses delegate and supervise the patient care activities of Licensed Practical Nurses and ancillary nursing personnel.

The nurse uses the nursing process to assess, plan, implement, and evaluate the plan of care, from admission assessment to discharge planning.

The nurse plans and provides care for each child/family that fulfills the criteria of the established nursing standards of CHMC. Registered nurses acknowledge, coordinate, and implement the diagnostic and therapeutic prescriptions of medical staff members.

Nursing services are integrated with the medical staff, and other disciplines that participate in patient care, through participation in mutual patient care conferences, mutual unit planning, Medical/Dental Staff committees, policy decisions, and institutional planning.

There are six major inpatient clinical services and three major outpatient clinical services providing nursing care at CHMC.

Section 1 Inpatient

A. **Pediatric Medical-Surgical Nursing Services**
   Each nurse maintains the knowledge and skills necessary to practice acute medical-surgical nursing.

B. **Pediatric Perioperative Care Nursing Services**
   Each nurse receives specialized training and/or orientation to perform pediatric surgical nursing care, and demonstrates and maintains the knowledge and skills necessary to care for patients in the pre-, inter-, and post-operative setting.

C. **Neonatal and Pediatric Critical Care Nursing Services**
   Each nurse, after an extensive period of orientation, demonstrates and maintains the skills and knowledge necessary for crisis intervention while caring for the patient in the critical care setting.

D. **Pediatric Chronic Care Nursing Services**
   Each nurse demonstrates and maintains the skills and knowledge necessary to care for the chronic patient over an extended period of time.

E. **Pediatric Rehabilitation Nursing Services**
   Each nurse demonstrates and maintains the knowledge and skills necessary to care for the patient during a specified period of rehabilitation.

F. **Pediatric Psychiatric Care Nursing Services**
   Each nurse, after an extensive period of orientation, maintains the knowledge and skills necessary for milieu management and behavior modification of the patient in the psychiatric setting.

Section 2 Outpatient

A. **Pediatric Emergency Care Nursing Services**
   Each nurse, after an extensive period of orientation, demonstrates and maintains the knowledge and skills necessary to practice emergency nursing, ranging from triage to trauma care, in the pediatric setting.

B. **Pediatric Ambulatory Care Nursing Services**
   Each nurse demonstrates and maintains the knowledge and skills necessary to perform general well-child nursing care, and/or care of a specific population in a designated speciality clinic or patient care area.

C. **Pediatric Home Health Care Nursing Services**
   Each nurse demonstrates and maintains the knowledge and skills necessary to educate, direct, and assist parents in caring for their child in the home setting, as well as providing episodic direct nursing care.

Section 3 Future services

Inpatient and outpatient nursing services may grow, change, or be added as the changing health care needs of patients and families are identified and addressed by CHMC.

IV. NURSING STAFF MEMBERSHIP

Membership on the nursing staff is a privilege that is extended to those who meet qualifications, standards and requirements as set forth in these articles.

Section 1   Qualifications for membership on the professional nursing staff

The professional nurse applicant for appointment to the nursing staff shall be legally licensed to practice nursing in the State of Ohio. This individual must meet all requirements and criteria indicated in these articles and agree to uphold and adhere to the requirements and conditions of these articles.

Section 2   Professional nursing staff membership

Professional membership is granted to those:

A. With the required nursing license to practice nursing in the State of Ohio.
B. Who can give evidence of required experience and education.
C. Who can demonstrate competence for the role.
D. Who adhere to the American Nursing Association Code of Ethics.
E. Who demonstrate the ability to interact with peers, patients/families, administration, and governance leadership.
F. Who have been approved by the process outlined in these articles and have had privileges granted.

No professional registered nurse is entitled to membership on the nursing staff or to the exercise of particular clinical nursing privileges in the hospital solely by the virtue of a license to practice in the State of Ohio without evidence of the above required qualifications.

Membership on the Professional Nurse Staff includes:
Clinical Nurse I
Clinical Nurse II
Clinical Nurse III
Clinical Nurse Specialists
Nurse Practitioners
Department Directors
Assistant Department Directors
Coordinators
Managers
Education Nurse Specialists
Clinical Nurse Researcher
Nursing Administrators

and others that will in the future be deemed appropriate by the Nursing Executive Council and who are privileged to practice within the context of these articles.

Professional nurses who are employed by CHMC, but outside the Division of Nursing, are eligible for Professional Nursing Staff membership.

The nurse must follow the credentialing and privileging process outlined in Article IV, Section 5. "Credentialing and Privileging Process."

In departments where there is no nurse manager, the obligations of that nurse manager position as identified in Section 5 shall be performed by a liaison professional nurse appointed by the Nursing Executive Council. In addition, the department manager must convey agreement in writing to the Nursing Quality Assurance Chairperson to membership of the professional nurses in the Professional Nursing Staff organization.

Section 3   Categories of other nursing memberships

Professional Nurses who are granted privileges in the following categories have the obligation to fulfil the responsibilities for which they are employed and are granted nursing staff privileges congruent with their assignment. They are not eligible to participate in the rights extended to the Professional Nursing Staff members.

A. **Consulting Nursing Staff**
   Consulting nursing staff privileges are granted to registered professional nurses duly licensed, who provide per diem consulting services to the nursing staff within the Division of Nursing.
   Application and approval of consulting privileges are obtained through the following procedure:
   1. Documentation of a current registered nurse license.
   2. Submission of applicants curriculum vitae.
   3. References/recommendations are obtained.
   4. Signing of a contract with the Vice President, Nursing.
   5. Consulting privileges applied for remain in force for no longer than 12 months from date of privilege acceptance and must be renewed following the above procedure.

B. **Agency Nursing Staff**
   Agency Nursing Staff privileges are granted to registered professional nurses who are employees of agencies which have a contract with the Division of Nursing and who have provided evidence of meeting the criteria outlined in the contract. Contracts will contain: licensing, experience and education, competence and health requirements for agency employees sent to CHMC and other criteria deemed necessary by the Division of Nursing. These professional nurses provide episodic nursing services within the Division of Nursing.
   Application and approval of agency privileges are obtained through the following procedure:
   1. The agency verifies that the employees of the agency have current licenses and meet the CHMC criteria of clinical competence in pediatric nursing.

2. The agency nurse completes two days of hospital orientation designed for the agency employee.

3. Agency nursing staff privileges are granted for the times the agency nurse is assigned to CHMC.

C. **Nurse Faculty Staff**

Faculty Nursing Staff privileges are granted to registered professional nurses who are employed by an academic institution which has a contractual agreement with CHMC and who are providing education and training to students utilizing the facility for educational services.

Contract criteria shall include defined health requirements, orientation requirements, agreement to adhere to CHMC policies and standards and other requirements which may be added to the school-CHMC contract in the future. Application and approval of Nurse Faculty Staff privileges are obtained through the following procedure:

1. Faculty are employed by schools or colleges of nursing who have a contract with CHMC.

2. Evidence is provided that the faculty members have completed the requirements of the contract.

3. Nurse Faculty Staff privileges are granted upon recommendation of the ESN staff member in charge of contracts.

D. **Temporary Nursing Staff**

Temporary Nursing Staff privileges are granted to registered professional nurses who are employed by the Division of Nursing of CHMC on a temporary basis as defined in CHMC Personnel Policy D-00 Categories of Employment.

Temporary privileges coincide with the term of employment.

Temporary privileges are defined by the employment agreement. Application and approval of Temporary Nursing Staff privileges are obtained through the following process:

1. Documentation of a current registered nurse license in Ohio.

2. Submission of applicant's curriculum vitae.

3. References/recommendations are obtained.

4. Signing of an employment agreement.

Section 4   Provisional nursing staff

A. The newly hired nurse is appointed as a provisional member of the nursing staff and is designated per unit or department. Failure to receive privileges to practice at professional status shall be deemed as termination from the nursing staff.

Provisional member status coincides with the CHMC Probationary Status. Provisional status and provisional privileges can be extended in accordance with the Human Resources Department policy #E-00, Probationary Evaluation.

B. Provisional nursing staff members are assigned to a department/unit where their performance is observed by a member of the professional nursing staff to determine eligibility for professional nursing staff membership.

C. Provisional nursing staff members are granted privileges for nursing practice appropriate to their demonstrated competence within their identified unit/department.

D. All provisional nursing staff members are granted the right to participate in a council, but do not have membership as identified within the context of these articles. They do not attain the right to vote or hold office.

Section 5   Credentialing and privileging process

A. **Credentials Review Process**

The credentials review process is an obligation of the Nursing Quality Assurance Council and is initiated and maintained for all professional nurse members. The process entails the review of the credentials of applicants to the nursing staff for membership.

1. The Quality Assurance Council invests responsibility in the CHMC Manager of Placement and Counseling for:

   a. review of all professional nurse applications for appropriateness of placement.

   b. review and acceptance of all credentials supplied by the applicants; i.e., nursing license in the State of Ohio, education, experience, certifications.

   c. completion of the employment process upon approval of the applicant from the unit/department manager.

2. The credentials review process consists of:

   a. Evidence that the applicant has the appropriate license, certificates or degrees, diplomas, or other evidence indicating required preparation.

   b. Completion of a successful interview for a nursing staff position with a nurse manager and a nurse peer. This step includes the verification of applicant's ability to be a resource to the unit/department, as well as the applicant's ability to uphold the nursing division's standards.

   c. Recommendation for approval by agreement of the nurse manager and nurse peer.

   d. Granting of provisional nursing staff privileges when requirements are met.

B. **Privilege Review Process**

The Privilege Review Process will be invested in the Nursing Quality Assurance Council.

The Privilege Review Process consists of:

1. Successful completion of the initial provisional privilege probationary time period.
2. The applicant's desire for professional privileges.
3. Petition by the unit/department manager and professional nurse peer on the behalf of the applicant, to the Nursing Quality Assurance Council.
4. Granting of Professional Nursing Staff Membership Privileges for the period of one year.
5. Yearly renewal of Professional Nursing Staff Membership Privileges based on a successful performance evaluation.

C. **Privileges to Advance Within the Clinical Advancement Program**
Membership of the Professional Nursing Staff may voluntarily apply for privileges within the Clinical Advancement Program. Applicants must successfully evidence achievement of identified standards for the level in which they apply.

D. **Appeals**
The Human Resource Department Conflict Resolution Process #F-07 is followed for appeals of the Clinical Advancement Program process.

Section 6   Rights obtained from professional nursing staff membership

Appointment to the Professional Nursing Staff confers on the appointee those clinical privileges which are within the level of nursing practice of their demonstrated competence. Professional Nursing Staff privileges are granted within the context of these articles and cannot be denied for any other reasons.

All members of the Professional Nursing Staff are granted the right and responsibility to participate in membership and vote within the designated councils as identified in the context of these articles. All members of the Professional Nursing Staff are granted the right to vote with the staff as a whole on matters pertaining to articles and election of the president.

Members of the Professional Nursing Staff whose position is 90% clinical are granted the right within the context of these articles to chair the Nursing Practice, Nursing Quality Assurance, Nursing Research, and Nursing Education Councils and other such bodies determined from time to time to be essential to the work of nursing.

Those members of the Professional Nursing Staff who hold management/administrative positions are granted the right to chair the Nursing Management Council.

Section 7   Obligations of the professional nursing staff

The application submitted for consideration within the Credential Review process constitutes the applicant's acknowledgement of staff obligations within the Professional Nursing Staff structure.

Appointment to the Professional Nursing staff confers on the nurse the clinical obligation to provide continuous nursing care of patients consistent with the standards of care and within the level of nursing practice of their demonstrated competence.

Members are obligated to participate in shared governance and to abide by the nursing staff articles and the rules and regulations of the Division of Nursing and to fulfill other such obligations that may be determined from time to time as essential by the Nursing Executive Council. Members are obligated to adhere to the values, standards and policies of CHMC.

V.   GOVERNANCE STRUCTURE
Section 1   Governance councils

There are five Governance Councils and an Executive Council that assume accountability for the management, operation and integration of the nursing division. The Governance Councils are identified as follows:

Nursing Practice Council

Nursing Education Council

Nursing Quality Assurance Council

Nursing Research Council

Nursing Management Council

Each Council is clearly identified in these articles and operates consistent with the mandates of its roles and accountabilities as defined in the articles.

Section 2   Council authority

These five Governance Councils are the legitimate formats for decision making in the division of nursing and retain the accountability for the process and outcome of all issues related to nursing practice, education, quality assurance, research and the management.

Section 3   Nursing practice council

A. **Role.** The Nursing Practice Council defines and controls all issues, materials and activities related to nursing practices reflective of shared governance and Rogerian theory.

B. **Accountabilities.** The Nursing Practice Council:
1. Develops, revises, implements and directs the clinical nursing standards including care, practice and performance and develops and implements nursing policies and procedures.
2. Represents nurses as an integral part of CHMC's interdisciplinary approach to patient care.

C. **Membership.** Membership on the Nursing Practice Council is drawn from the professional nursing staff with two representatives selected from each cluster. (See Rules and Regulations for identification). Representatives have the acceptance of the Council. The

Chairperson meets the specific requirements for the position and is elected from the voting council membership. Other members are:

1. One Clinical Nurse Specialist
2. One Nurse Practitioner
3. One Nursing Management Council representative

Additional members can be added from time to time by majority vote for a period of time as deemed necessary by the work of the Council.

Section 4   Nursing education council

A. **Role.** The Nursing Education Council defines and evaluates nursing education needs within the Division of Nursing for the purpose of developing a highly skilled nursing staff that provides quality patient care.
B. **Accountabilities.** The Nursing Education Council:
   1. Promulgates education within the Division of Nursing.
   2. Establishes and maintains an effective communication system.
   3. Coordinates the quarterly and annual staff meetings.
C. **Membership.** Membership on the Nursing Education Council is drawn from the professional nursing staff with two representatives selected from each cluster. (See Rules and Regulations for identification). The Chairperson meets the specific requirements for the position and is elected from the voting council membership. Other members are:
   1. One Education Nurse Specialist
   2. One Nursing Management Council representative

Additional members can be added from time to time by majority vote of the council for a period of time as deemed necessary by the work of the council.

Section 5   Nursing quality assurance council

A. **Role.** The Nursing Quality Assurance Council designs, structures and implements the Division of Nursing's quality improvement program leading to improved patient care and maintains the Division of Nursing's Privileging and Credentialing process.
B. **Accountabilities.** The Nursing Quality Assurance Council:
   1. Establishes a divisional quality assurance plan that is unit-based in focus and philosophy and ensures that the unit-based implementation of the plan is operational.
   2. Undertakes problem identification and corrective action to improve patient care.
   3. Integrates the nursing quality assurance program with hospital quality assurance systems to detect trends and patterns of performance that effect more than one department or service.
   4. Evaluates the effectiveness of the quality assurance program consistent with or exceeding the requirements of regulatory agencies.
   5. Assists in the evaluation of programs within the Division of Nursing.
   6. Ensures the quality of the professional nurse providing nursing care through the credentialing and privileging process and the evaluation of candidates for clinical advancement.
C. **Membership.** Membership on the Nursing Quality Assurance Council is drawn from the professional nursing staff with one representative selected from each cluster. The Chairperson meets the specific requirements for the position and is elected from the voting Council membership. Other members are:
   1. One Nursing Management Council representative

Additional members can be added from time to time by majority vote of the council for a period of time as deemed necessary by the work of the Council.

Section 6   Nursing research council

A. **Role.** The Nursing Research Council validates knowledge upon which nursing practice is based and generates new knowledge to advance the science and practice of nursing through the promotion and support of nursing research.
B. **Accountabilities.** The Nursing Research Council:
   1. Develops, maintains and evaluates a nursing research program in collaboration with the nurse researcher.
   2. Manages and assists in the generation of nursing research funds.
   3. Facilitates education of Division of Nursing members on the value and the process of nursing research and utilization of research findings.
   4. Establishes liaisons with researchers and organizations related to nursing and child/family health research at the local, state, national and international level for the purpose of promoting change in the practice of nursing at CHMC and elsewhere.
C. **Membership.** Membership on the Nursing Research Council is drawn from the professional nursing staff with one council representative selected from each cluster. The Chairperson meets the specific requirements for the position and is elected from the voting Council membership. Other members are:
   1. Clinical Nurse Researcher
   2. One Nursing Management Council representative

Additional members can be added from time to time by majority vote for a period of time as deemed necessary by the work of the Council.

Section 7 Nursing management council

A. **Role.** The Nursing Management Council organizes and controls resources, delineates and fulfills nursing management objectives and develops an environment that promotes and enhances the practice of professional nursing.

B. **Accountabilities.** The Nursing Management Council manages, controls and allocates the following resources:

1. Human. Providing the appropriate human resources necessary to meet the standards of practice in all areas of care.
2. Fiscal. Development of a budgetary philosophy reflective of the current economic environment.
3. Operational Systems. Determine systems that support management.
4. Support. Assume the accountability for carrying out the mandates of the nursing organization from the governance councils by ensuring that the council decisions are communicated and implemented.
5. Materials. Providing the material resources necessary to meet patient care requirements.

C. Membership on the Nursing Management Council is drawn from the professional nursing staff holding management positions within the Division of Nursing and a representative from the clinical professional nursing staff. Each category of management represented determines the selection process for their representative. Not more than two representatives will come from a unit. The chairperson meets the specific requirements for the position and is elected from the voting council membership. Members are:

1. Vice President
2. One Assistant Vice President
3. Four Department Directors
4. Two Assistant Department Directors
5. One Manager, Patient Services
6. One Clinical Nurse Representative

Additional members can be added from time to time by majority vote of the council for the period of time deemed necessary by the work of the council.

Section 8 Selection of governance council membership

Members of the governance councils are selected from the designated clusters, clinical services or management roles. Staff council representative are chosen from each cluster on a rotating basis. Each unit determines the selection process for the representative to their cluster. Each group represented in other members category, determines the selection process for their representative of the council. All units assume responsibility for membership when it is their turn on the rotation. Each council shall have representatives from a variety of services. Representatives to the staff councils must hold positions which are ninety percent clinical practice or be unit education coordinators. Representative council members serve two year terms. Half of the council's membership changes yearly in January. If a representative is unable to complete their term, a replacement from the same unit completes the term. Members can be reappointed to the same council after an absence of one year.

Section 9 Service of council members

Members are required to attend eighty percent of all scheduled council meetings. During any absences from staff councils, an alternate attends. Alternates for Nursing Management Council are designated by the represented group for absences of more than three meetings.

Section 10 Council committees

All council committees have specific objectives, focus and time frames. The committees report to the council Chairperson at least quarterly and are reviewed at least annually regarding their purpose and continuance. There are a maximum of three committees per council. One third of total membership of the committee constitutes a quorum. One council member sits on the committee and serves as a liaison to the council. The council approves the committee's Chairperson. The council retains final authority for all committee recommendations.

Section 11 Meetings

All governance councils meet at least monthly and are responsible for the work of each council consistent with these articles. Minutes are taken and duly recorded in the approved governance format. One half plus one of the total representatives of the Council constitutes a quorum and is deemed appropriate for conducting the business of the Council.

VI. OFFICERS OF THE NURSING STAFF ORGANIZATION

The officers of the Nursing staff are the President and the Chairs of the Councils.

A. **Chairs of Councils**

1. Qualifications. The chairperson of the staff councils is a professional nurse whose position is ninety percent clinical. The chairperson of the Management Council is a professional nurse who holds a management position within the Nursing Division.
2. Elections. Each governance council has in place a mechanism for electing their chairperson-elect, which takes place in November. The chairperson-elect serves a one year term at the end of which they assume the role of chairperson.
3. Term. The term of office is from January 1 to De-

cember 31 of the year following the election. The chairperson may not serve consecutive years and is not eligible for a chairperson-elect position on any council for one year following the term. Council membership ends when the chairperson's term has expired. During their term, the chairperson does not represent any constituency.

4. Vacancies. If the chairperson is unable to assume or complete the term of the position, the chairperson-elect assumes the chairperson position. If the chairperson-elect is unable to assume or complete the term of the position, the nominee who received the second highest number of votes assumes the position. The election results and ballots are maintained for one year from the time of the election by the Vice President, Nursing.

5. Powers of the Chair. The chair of each governance council assures the accountabilities of their council are fulfilled. The chair represents the council and acts on its behalf; the chair mediates and arbitrates disagreements between unit and divisional councils and between managers and staff within their areas of accountability; the chair removes representatives who are not fulfilling their responsibilities.

B. **President**

1. President of the Nursing Staff. Qualified nominees for the position are selected from staff members who have been active members of a divisional council for the previous year.

2. Election of the President of the Nursing Staff. A nominating committee, comprised of (one) representative from each staff council and the outgoing President develop the application and election process. The election is decided by a majority vote of the professional nursing staff who vote.

3. Term of the President of the Nursing Staff. The President is elected for a term of one year which runs from January 1st to December 31st of the year following the election.

4. Vacancies of the office of President of the Nursing Staff. If unable to assume or complete the terms of the position, the nominee receiving the second highest number of the votes assumes the position. The election results and ballots are maintained for (one) year by the Vice President, Nursing.

5. Powers of the President of the Nursing Staff. The President of the Nursing Staff assures the accountabilities of the Nursing Executive Council are fulfilled. The President represents the council and the Professional Nursing Organization and acts on its behalf; the President removes nursing council chairs who are not fulfilling their responsibilities; the chair works collaboratively with the Vice President, Nursing in implementing the articles.

VII. DISCIPLINE, APPEALS, AND REMOVAL

Section 1 Discipline, appeals, and removal from the nursing staff

All members of the nursing staff, regardless of their position, are subject to the personnel standards and discipline policies of CHMC Human Resources Department. All members of the nursing staff are entitled to and protected by the grievance process as detailed in the personnel policy on Conflict Resolution. (# F-07 Personnel Policy.)

When a member of the nursing staff fails to perform the duties stated in their position description, or to uphold the standards of the Division of Nursing or the institution, they may be disciplined or removed from the staff and their privileges to practice nursing within the institution revoked.

The nurse manager is responsible for initiating the disciplinary and/or removal process for a professional nurse as outlined in Personnel Policy F-05 (Employee Discipline).

The professional nurse has the right to dispute disciplinary actions related to professional practice and has the right to utilize the formal process to have a grievance objectively reviewed. The CHMC policy will be followed with the following exception made within the Conflict Resolution Committee. The committee will be chosen as follows.

> The affected nurse chooses the chairperson from four management employees who are initially appointed to the committee status by the President, CHMC.
>
> The chairperson then confirms a second committee member who will be a Nursing Practice Council member from the nurses department and has been chosen by the Chair of The Division of Nursing Practice Council. The grieving employee must agree to this selection.
>
> The nurse will select the third committee member from the Professional Nursing Staff. The chairperson must agree to the grieving employee's selection.

Section 2 Discipline, appeals, and removal from the governance structure

A. **Councils.** The Shared Governance Councils are responsible for decisions regarding their accountabilities. These decisions are not grievable. Shared Governance issues are not grievable through the Conflict Resolution Policy of the CHMC Human Resources Department.

B. **Unit Councils.** Each unit is responsible for addressing concerns regarding performance of duties. Each unit is responsible for having procedures for removal and replacement of members on their unit councils.

C. **Council Representatives.** Concerns regarding a council representative's performance of duties should be addressed directly to the representative by the individual council member having the concern. If unresolved, the concerns will be addressed by the Review Group (nominating committee), who will make recommendations to the Chair.

The Chair is responsible for removal of a representative.

D. **Council Chair-elect.** Concerns regarding the Chairelect's performance of duties should be addressed directly to the Chair-elect by the individual council member having the concern. If unresolved, the concerns should be addressed to the following (in order):

1. Chair of the specific council.
2. Review Group (nominating committee), who will make recommendations to the Chair.

   The Chair is responsible for removal of the Chairelect.

E. **Council Chair.** Concerns regarding the Chair's performance of duties should be addressed directly to the Chair by the individual member of the council having the concern. If unresolved, the concerns should be addressed to the following (in order):

1. Assistant Vice President advisor
2. Review Group (nominating committee), who will make recommendations to the Chair.
3. Executive Council Chair

   The Executive Council Chair is responsible for removal of the Council Chair.

F. **President of the Nursing Staff (Executive Council Chair).** Concerns regarding the President's performance of duties should be addressed directly to the President by the individual member of the staff having the concern. If unresolved, the concerns should be addressed to the following (in order):

1. Vice President, Nursing
2. Review Group (nominating committee of the staff), who will make recommendation to the Executive Council.
3. Executive Council.

   Executive Council is responsible for removal of the President of the Nursing Staff.

G. **Appeals.** Grievances that arise within the Shared Governance structure should be addressed in the following manner:

1. The individual discusses the issues with the Manager of Nursing Recruitment and Retention.
2. The appellant formally files a grievance with the Manager of Nursing Recruitment and Retention.
3. A review panel comprised of the President of Nursing Staff plus one member from each council, ex-

cluding the council to which the nurse filing the grievance was a member, hears all pertinent information and arrives at a decision. If consensus is not achieved, decision will be by majority vote.

VIII. COORDINATION OF THE NURSING DIVISION

Section 1 Administration

The Vice President, Nursing is responsible and accountable to the Executive Vice President/Chief Operating Officer, the Chief Executive Officer/Medical Chief of Staff and the Board of Trustees of Children's Hospital Medical Center for the coordination, integration and administration of the Division of Nursing and the clinical nursing services provided. In this role, the Vice President, Nursing Services: assures that the articles, rules and regulations, policies and procedures promulgated by the nursing staff organization are enforced. The Vice President also integrates the activities of the nursing staff organization and the institution as a whole.

The Assistant Vice President, Nursing provides administrative direction to designated patient units, nursing projects and programs. This role functions as an extension of the Vice President, Nursing.

Section 2 Nursing executive council

A. **Role.** The Nursing Executive Council integrates the governance structure within the Division of Nursing and ensures its effective operation.

B. **Accountabilities.** The Nursing Executive Council.

1. Integrates the mission, values and goals of CHMC into all aspects of the Shared Governance structure.
2. Maintains the Shared Governance structure including development, revision and control of the articles and the rules and regulations.
3. Coordinates the work of the Divisional Councils.

C. **Membership.** Membership on the Nursing Executive Council is comprised of the Chairpersons of the five governance councils the President of the Nursing Staff and the Vice President, Nursing. The President of the Nursing Staff serves as the Chairperson of the Nursing Executive Council. The members of the Nursing Executive Council are the officers of the nursing staff.

Section 3 Meetings

A. **Executive Council.** The Nursing Executive Council meets at least monthly and is responsible for the work delineated within these articles. Minutes are taken and duly recorded in the approved governance format. One half plus one of the total representatives of the council constitutes a quorum and is deemed appropriate for conducting the business of the Council.

B. **Annual and Quarterly Professional Nursing Staff Meetings.** The annual meeting includes the review of the nursing division's goals, activities of the governance councils, the announcement of the elected President of the Nursing Staff and any other business as identified on the agenda. The professional nursing staff also meets at least quarterly. The purpose of the quarterly meetings is to review and approve the business of the nursing staff as presented by the Nursing Executive Council. On matters submitted for a staff vote, a majority of members present is sufficient for passing with the exception of the articles which require a 2/3 majority vote. The meeting is chaired by the President of the Nursing Staff who conducts the meeting according to *Robert's Rules of Order*. Issues and motions from the staff can be addressed in this meeting following their review and approval for addition to the agenda by the Chairperson.

Section 4   Management

A. Directors. The Director facilitates, coordinates and integrates the work of unit councils and ensures their effective operation within the shared governance structure. The Director is responsible and accountable for providing input to the councils on available resources and for controlling the allocation of these resources. The Director integrates the unit with hospital systems to meet patient care requirements and employee needs.

B. Assistant Directors. Assists the Director in providing nursing management leadership. The Assistant Director assumes the responsibility within the unit for facilitating and coordinating patient care delivery, effective communication and staff growth and development.

C. Manager, Patient Services. The Manager, Patient Services is the nursing divisional manager weekday evenings and nights, weekends and holidays. The Manager functions as an extension of the role of the Department Director as appropriate for the issue. They act as a liaison between nursing, other departments and in-house services during their assigned shift.

Section 5   Physicians

The nursing professional organization and its structure is integrated with the Medical/Dental Professional Staff organization and its structures to address patient care issues. An interdisciplinary, collaborative relationship provides the patient and family with the required level of service.

Section 6   Administrative advisor role on divisional council

A. **Qualifications**
   1. Assistant Vice President
   2. Appointed by Vice President

B. **Tenure**
   1. The term of assignment will be one year from July 1 to June 30.
C. **Vacancies**
   In the event of a vacancy, the Vice President will appoint a replacement.
D. **Responsibilities**
   1. Assist Chair and Chair-elect in development of skills
   2. Meet monthly with chair to assist in the development of the agenda and coordination of the council
   3. Serve as a resource to the Chair and members of the council regarding hospital strategic planning policies, organizational purposes and mission divisional policies and regulatory requirements
   4. Act as an extension of the Vice President
   5. Integrate the councils with the division and the hospital
   6. Provide a broad divisional and hospital perspective
   7. Ensure that the interest, decisions, and concerns of the council are represented in other forums (hospital, community)

IX.   ARTICLE REVISION
Section 1   Amendments

The articles of the nursing staff may be amended at any quarterly meeting of the professional nursing staff. Any professional nursing staff member may recommend changes in the articles by submitting their recommendations to council Divisional Chairperson. The council Chairperson presents the proposed article change to the Nursing Executive Council for review and at their discretion, inclusion on the agenda of the next regularly scheduled professional nursing staff meeting. The proposed amendments are published and made available to the professional nursing staff for review and consideration 6 weeks prior to the next regularly scheduled staff meeting. A two-thirds majority vote of the professional nursing staff attending the next regularly scheduled staff meeting is required for adoption. Revised articles are presented to the Board of Trustees for review and approval.

X.   ADOPTION

These articles are adopted at the annual professional nursing staff meeting by a two-thirds majority of the members voting. They shall replace any previous articles and are subject to the mandates and approval of the hospital Board of Trustees.

———————————————   ———————————————
Chair, Board of Trustees   C.O.O.

———————————————   ———————————————
Vice President, Nursing   President of Nursing Staff

RULES AND REGULATIONS

RULES AND REGULATIONS

The nursing staff, through its constituent councils, adopts such rules and regulations as are necessary to implement and maintain these articles from time to time based on need. All new or changed rules and regulations are approved by the Executive Council prior to their implementation. Such changes are effective upon approval of the Executive Council.

Section 1   Nursing executive council

A. Responsibilities
1. Formulation, coordination, dissemination and evaluation of yearly Nursing Division goals.
2. Development and revision of articles for the nursing staff organization governance.
3. Yearly recommendations regarding nursing staff members to Medical/Dental Staff committees and hospital committees.
4. Coordination of the work of the divisional councils, including mediation of disputes.
5. Implementation of the shared governance structure and evaluation of its effectiveness, including discipline as necessary.

B. Member Responsibilities
1. Represent the council in other forums.
2. Provide information to the council from the governance councils.
3. Communicate the business of the council to the governance council's membership on a regular basis.

Section 2   Nursing practice council

A. Responsibilities
1. Develop and revise a professional practice model.
2. Develop and implement nursing practice programs.
3. Resolve identified nursing practice issues and problems.
4. Integrate an identified conceptual framework in all areas of nursing practice.

5. Incorporate research findings into nursing practice.
6. Function as a resource regarding nursing practice issues both internally and externally.
7. Mediate and arbitrate conflicts between council and unit councils and between unit councils and managers.
8. Develop and revise a framework for guidelines for unit practice councils.
9. Define the scope of responsibilities of LPNs and ancillary nursing care providers.
10. Develop and/or approve nursing documentation standards and forms.
11. Assist in the development of hospital and medical/dental staff clinical policies and procedures.
12. Participate in clinical focused interdisciplinary problem solving and program development.
13. Function as nursing clinical consultants to other groups.
14. Seek input and interdisciplinary collaboration on appropriate clinical practices issues.
15. Represent clinical nursing on the appropriate Medical/Dental Staff committees.
16. Refer and consult with Nursing Management Council on identified issues.
17. Refer QA and education needs based on practice decisions.
18. Assess and recommend modifications of systems which impact nursing practice.

B. Member Responsibilities
1. Represent the council in other forums.
2. Serve as a resource to the units concerning practice issues.
3. Elicit input from units, represent unit concerns, needs and desires.
4. Make decisions based on the best possible outcome for the whole (patient, hospital, unit, peers, etc.).
5. Communicate in a timely manner goals, actions, decisions and rationale to the unit representatives.
6. Assure decisions of council are implemented.
7. Perform duties as assigned.

C. Designated Committees:
1. Standards Committee
2. Computer Committee
3. Conceptual Framework Committee

Section 3   Nursing quality assurance council

A. Responsibilities
1. Monitor and evaluate the quality and appropriateness of patient care delivered through structure, process and outcome measurement.
2. Identify patient care improvement opportunities.
3. Recognize and promote the need for continuous quality improvement.

4. Recommend and/or implement action plans in a timely manner. When not in compliance, see that corrective action takes place at the division and unit level.

5. Evaluate action plans through ongoing monitoring and evaluation at the division and unit level.

6. Ensure demonstration and maintenance of acceptable levels of qualified clinical competency and appropriate credentialing and privileging of all professional nurses based on position descriptions and criteria based performance evaluations.

7. Communicate to the Vice President Nursing information regarding the quality review of nursing roles at CHMC.

8. Assure that pertinent findings from nursing and patient care monitoring and evaluations are disseminated to involved nurses throughout the Division of Nursing.

9. Integrate quality assurance with the goals and objectives of the Nursing Division, as well as the philosophy of CHMC.

10. Supply monthly quality assurance minutes and quarterly reports to the hospital quality assurance committee.

11. Set annual priorities based on those of the Nursing Executive Council.

12. Provide member of the division with opportunities and mechanisms for advancement through peer review and the clinical advancement program.

B. **Member Responsibilities**

1. Assist units with follow through of the QA plan and proper record keeping information.

2. Communicate to the units/departments all information needed from council meetings to implement our QA program.

3. Reports to council any cluster activities concerns and issues.

4. Update cluster membership quarterly.

5. Serve as a resource for Division of Nursing Quality Assurance program.

6. Perform duties as assigned.

7. Provide positive role modeling for Quality Assurance.

8. Make decisions based on the best possible outcome for the division as a whole.

9. Assure council decisions are implemented.

10. Cluster representative will serve as unit representatives with the exception of the chair.

C. **QA Representative Meetings**

1. Quarterly the QA representatives from all units in the Division of Nursing shall meet with the QA Council for the purpose of education and dissemination of information.

2. Each unit will be responsible to select their own representative.

D. **Designated Committees:**

1. Clinical Advancement Committee

2. Credentialing Committee

Section 4 Education council

A. **Responsibilities**

1. Develop educational goals for the Division of Nursing.

2. Ascertain common educational needs of nursing staff.

3. Design and coordinate programs to meet common learning needs of nursing.

4. Improve the quality of nursing care by offering staff educational programs.

5. Coordinate the interpretation and development of nursing orientation objectives on a hospital wide and unit based level utilizing available resources.

6. Maintain a communication system which will consist of (a) weekly newsletter, (b) concise minute format, (c) council agenda referral tool, and (d) bi-annual nursing magazine and any tool that may be necessary from time to time.

7. Provide communication and facilitate education on new or revised practice and technologies.

8. Aid Education Council members in developing effective methods to communicate information to unit nursing personnel.

9. Communicate planned unit inservices, conferences, workshops, seminars, orientation and other educational opportunities to council members.

10. Evaluate educational programs within the Division of Nursing.

11. Determine guidelines for management and distribution of educational monies from the continuing education funds.

B. **Member Responsibilities**

1. Represent the council in other forums.

2. Serve as role models and facilitators for education and professional development.

3. Elicit input from the units, represent unit concerns, needs and desires.

4. Make decisions based upon the best possible outcomes for the whole (patient, hospital, unit, peers, etc.)

5. Communicate in a timely manner goals, actions, decisions and rationale to unit representatives.

6. Assure implementation of council decisions.

7. Perform duties as assigned.

8. Cluster representatives will serve as unit representatives with the exception of the chair and chair-elect.

C. **Designated Committees:**

1. Nursing Grand Rounds Committee

2. Perioperative Education Committee

Section 5   Nursing research council

A. **Responsibilities:**
   1. Establish nursing research priorities for the Division of Nursing.
   2. Serve as a resource for conducting nursing research and utilizing findings within the Division of Nursing.
   3. Grant approval for nursing research to be conducted within the Division of Nursing prior to Institutional Review Board Review.
   4. Appropriate monies from the nursing research funds.
   5. Facilitate and coordinate the communication of nursing research findings within the Division of Nursing.
   6. Promote nurses' participation in workshops, conferences and organizations focused on nursing research.

B. **Member Responsibilities:**
   1. Represent the council in other forms.
   2. Serve as a facilitator for the generation, communication and use of nursing research and findings on units within their cluster group.
   3. Elicit input from and represent unit cluster group concerns, needs and desires.
   4. Make decisions based on the best possible outcome for the whole (patient, hospital, unit, peers, etc.).
   5. Communicate in a timely manner goals, actions, decisions and rationale to cluster group unit representatives.
   6. Ensure decisions of the council are implemented.
   7. Perform duties and tasks assigned.
   8. Cluster representatives will serve as unit representatives with the exception of the chair and chair-elect.

C. **Research Representative Meetings.**
   1. Quarterly Research Council representatives from all the units in the Division of Nursing will meet with the Research Council for the purpose of education and dissemination of information and/or research findings.
   2. Each unit is be responsible for selecting their own representative.

D. **Designated Committees:**
   1. Funding Award Committee
   2. Proposal Review Committee

Section 6   Nursing management council

A. **Responsibilities**
   1. Determine appropriate staff mix and levels.
   2. Define non-clinical roles of nursing personnel.
   3. Determine standards of practice for non-clinical nursing personnel.
   4. Determine standards of practice for management personnel.
   5. Develop and evaluate incentive programs.
   6. Develop, implement and evaluate recruitment and retention programs.
   7. Determine nursing budget philosophy and priorities within a financial framework that is responsive to the changing economic environment.
   8. Participate in the development of divisional budgeting process.
   9. Review quarterly fiscal reports.
   10. Develop and coordinate implementation of nursing management policies.
   11. Determine management support systems.
   12. Interface with hospital systems to facilitate resolution of operational problems.
   13. Provide resource support for other councils' decisions and programs.
   14. Recommend management development programs.
   15. Ensure appropriate physical environment.
   16. Facilitate and promote a clinical power base in which employees may enhance their professional and personal growth.
   17. Ensure provision of equipment and supplies.
   18. Serve as a role model and teacher for the staff in their development as leaders in the shared governance system.
   19. Provide the strategic planning necessary to provide the environment that promotes and enhances the practice of professional nursing.

B. **Member Responsibilities**
   1. Represent the council in other forums.
   2. Serve as a resource to the units concerning resource issues.
   3. Provide information to the council from the representative group.
   4. Make decisions based on the best possible outcome for the whole.
   5. Communicate the business of the council to the represented groups on a regular basis.
   6. Serve as an active participant on the staff councils in order to provide support for the council's resource needs.
   7. Ensure that council decisions are implemented, followed up and action is taken on the unit level.
   8. Perform duties as assigned.

C. **Designated Committee:**
   Recruitment and Retention Committee

Section 7   Chair duties responsibilities

A. Screen incoming requests and issues, develop council meeting agendas, chair council meetings and call for a vote if consensus is not reached.
B. Delegate council assignments.
C. Remove representatives who are not fulfilling their responsibilities.

D. Make decisions when necessary on behalf of the council and communicate decisions at the next scheduled meeting.
E. Initiate or approve emergency meetings.
F. Represent council at Executive Council meetings.
G. Represent council at other forums and meet regularly with Assistant Vice President/Vice President advisor to review, plan, and receive advice.
H. Review the council's activities and adherence to the council's purpose, plans and goals.
I. In the event that the unit Coordination Council and the manager cannot reach a decision, the divisional council chair who owns accountability for the stated problem becomes the mediator, then arbitrator, then makes the final decision.

Section 8 Chair-elect responsibilities

A. General Responsibilities
1. Signs minutes and ensures distribution.
2. Performs duties and responsibilities of Chair in Chair's absence.
3. Assists Chair in planning, communicating and setting agenda.
4. Assumes responsibilities of Chair if position is vacated.

B. Council Specific Responsibilities
1. Practice Council
   Represents Practice Council at meeting of the Clinical Practice Committee (Medical/Dental staff).
2. Quality Assurance Council
   Represents Nursing Quality Assurance Council at the Hospital QA Committee (2 year term).

Section 9 Clustering

Clusters are identified groupings of departments/units.

Each department/unit sends a representative to their cluster group.

The cluster group members represent their cluster on the divisional councils.

Within the group, the cluster group members will determine council assignments.

The identified clusters are:

1	2	3
Emergency Department	3 South	3 East
4 West	3 West	4 East
Transport	Dialysis	2 East
CCU	NST	CRC
ICU		

4	5	6
4C West	PACU	2 South
4C North	OR	2 West
4C East	OPN	1 South
4C Trach	TC #5	SRU
4C PU/BU	OPS	
	OPD	

Section 10 Meetings

All Councils will meet routinely. Meeting times and places are designated in the official publication of Nursing Division. All meetings are open to observation with prior notification of the Chair. Council meeting times are:

A. Nursing Practice Council
   1. Fourth Thursday of every month.
B. Quality Assurance Council
   1. Fourth Wednesday of every month.
   2. Quarterly (2nd Wednesday of January, April, July, October) the representatives from all units/departments shall meet with the council for the purpose of education and dissemination of information.
C. Research Council
   1. Second Thursday of every month.
   2. Quarterly (2nd Thursday of March, June, September, December).
D. Education Council
   1. First Tuesday of every month.
E. Management Council
   1. First and third Tuesday of every month.
F. Executive Council
   1. Third Wednesday of every month.

Staff meetings quarterly in March, June, September and December. December meeting is the annual meeting.

Index

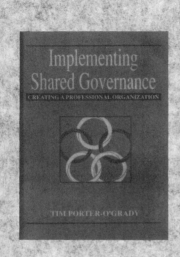
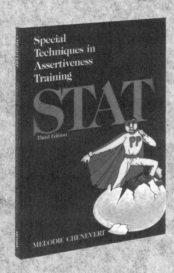
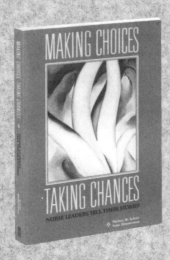